Grade *A* Baby Eggs

An Infertility Memoir

Grade A Baby Eggs

An Infertility Memoir

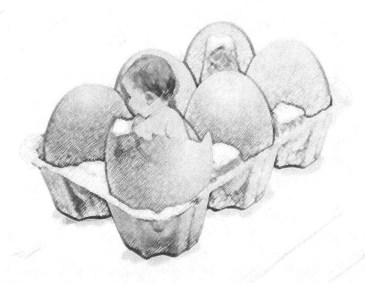

Victoria Hopewell

EPIGRAPH BOOKS
RHINEBECK, NY

Book and cover design by Joe Tantillo.

Epigraph Books
22 East Market Street, Suite 304
Rhinebeck, New York 12572
www.epigraphPS.com
USA 845-876-4861

ISBN 978-1-9369401-1-0
Library of Congress Control Number: 2011932259

Author's Note: The names of all the people mentioned in *Grade A Baby Eggs*, including the author, have been changed to protect their privacy. There also have been changes in identifying information.

To my family

Contents

Chapter One

Delusions of Eggdeur

The two-inch-long needle gleamed in the lamplight. It was suspended in midair. Beneath the needle lay my exposed buttocks. I was sprawled across the bed.

I clenched the mattress as I awaited impact. I pictured the syringe soaring through the sky. Then it began to lose altitude. It went into a tailspin. The pilot, my husband, lost control, and the plane crashed into my rear. I felt immediate pain.

"Victoria, that wasn't so bad. It was just a little bee sting. Buzz, buzz," said my husband, Gabriel.

"What are you talking about? It was a 747 that landed."

My husband reached for the first-aid kit. He swabbed alcohol over my wound, applied hot compresses, and massaged my butt cheek. Next I rolled over to start again. This time the needle would stab my stomach.

After six months of marriage, my husband and I had not resorted to S&M foreplay. This was not a sexual fantasy where he was a jet pilot and my bare butt was the landing strip, nor was he dressed as a bumblebee. Rather we just were following doctor's orders. We were trying to create a baby.

Our doctor was a renowned baby maker. My husband and I were informed consumers, and we had chosen a premier research physician from a topnotch New York hospital.

At the first appointment, the doctor lightly shook two of my fingers, looked up at the ceiling without making eye contact, and told me to sit down. I did not care that his patient skills were minimal. I just wanted him to get me pregnant. Gabriel could not take time off from work, so it was just me.

I felt privileged to be sitting in the doctor's office. I had needed to qualify for the hospital "fertility club" before I was even granted this meeting.

When I first called the hospital, the receptionist was skeptical.

"At forty-four you probably don't have the numbers. You can't make your own baby without those lower numbers."

"What do you mean? What numbers?" I asked.

"You need a blood test first. Your FSH—follicle-stimulating hormone—must be under 12. Of course we prefer lower than 9. Your estrogen level has to be under 70. At your age you could easily be perimenopausal. Then all your numbers would be too high."

"Well, can I at least find out?"

"You need to come in after your period. Then we'll know."

My levels were phenomenal. My FSH was 6 and my estrogen was 28. The results made me the Ponce de León of the fertility fountain of youth. I might not have the flawless, wrinkle-free skin to put me on an Oil of Olay commercial. Hormonally, however, I was as young as they come.

Now I proudly cited my numbers to the doctor.

"My levels are so great, I'm sure they'll be no problem in my getting pregnant."

"Actually your chances of pregnancy are in the single digits."

"What are you talking about?"

"The problem's your age. The chances of getting pregnant in your forties are very slim."

"But surely there are plenty of pregnant forty-year-olds."

"Not really. Biology takes over. A good example is the study of women in a religious sect in the Midwest. They did not believe in utilizing birth control. In their twenties and thirties they produced large families. However, even without contraception, they stopped having babies in their forties. This illustrates my point that women become incapable of getting pregnant as they become older."

"But certainly IVF will help me."

"You can't change biology. You are born with all of your eggs. No new eggs are created. By the time you're in your forties your eggs are no longer of the same quality. Indeed the odds are higher that the eggs will become genetically defective. Sperm, on the other hand, are produced on a regular basis. Therefore, the man can father children even when much older."

I was cornered. This wasn't even a mutual problem. It was *my* age and *my* elderly eggs that were at fault.

The doctor smiled for the first time. "You should consider egg donation. Your best chance is to use the eggs of someone in her twenties or early thirties."

He went on pleasantly about the hospital's excellent egg donor program, saying that he could get me material about it and that I could utilize the egg of a student from a local college or affiliated medical school.

My response was immediate. "I want to use my own egg. I have a great FSH level, and my husband and I want to try IVF with my egg and his sperm!"

The doctor backed off. "Fine," he said. However, he had to caution me that the odds would be much higher with a donor egg. I said that I would take my chances.

How could the doctor suggest that I use another woman's egg? The whole point was to have my own baby. Why would I want someone else's? I felt as though I was being expelled from the fertility sorority right after I joined. The receptionist had been wrong about my likely perimenopausal hormone level. I would prove the doctor wrong too.

I had practice beating the odds. I was lucky enough to marry Gabriel.

When I became a divorcée at age thirty-nine with four- and six-year-old daughters, the chance of remarriage was poor. Yet I overcame the probability statistics and found a husband five years later. But I was proactive. I engaged in singles activities rather than just waiting for a husband to arrive.

The most unusual one was Date Bait: sixty seconds to sell yourself at Manhattan's 92nd Street Y, a Jewish community and cultural center. In sixty seconds you had to stand up and provide a commercial with yourself as the product. As a Date Bait regular, I had perfected the right way to talk. It was important not to start sweating profusely, begin stammering, or collapse into the chair after stating your name. At the end of the event there were "matches" based on men and women mutually picking each other. Two different times I was told by the organizer that I was the lucky highest-scoring match person! I must still look young if I was chosen a lot—plus some of the matches were with younger men. This gave me confidence that I must be physically fit for baby production.

Gabriel was not one of my Date Bait catches. We met twice at different singles gatherings. The initial event, at a restaurant, started with hors d'oeuvres and talk with prospective singles. Then, in case that part wasn't going well, there was a diversion: we could watch a comedian perform.

My future husband came over and started talking with me during the first five minutes of hors d'oeuvres. The conversation never stopped. We compared the merits of different singles organizations. I was relatively new to the singles world, but Gabriel was much more knowledgeable. He'd had years of firsthand experience with dating options. He had even taken singles trips to exotic places like Costa Rica. He also knew the best charity events for meeting people, such as the Multiple Sclerosis annual gala.

Next we discussed Charleston, South Carolina. Gabriel went to school there and knew the interesting places to visit. I had always wanted to visit Charleston.

Meanwhile the "comedy phase" had begun. The female comedian was standing in a corner of the room making jokes over a microphone. We continued talking and became the butt of her jokes: she wondered how our "first date" was progressing and if we'd be a successful statistic. Gabriel and I didn't care. We were happy to have met.

At the end of the night came the moment of truth. I confided that I was not only divorced but that I had two children. Most men heard "children" and immediately stated that they couldn't see me. Gabriel still scribbled my phone number. I was hopeful. However, he never called.

Not being one to sit by the phone waiting, I dated other people and forgot about Gabriel. There still was no one special. Three years later I was at a huge singles party at a bar. There were no comforting activities: it was just a "thrown into the lions' den" type of event, with a thousand people who all belonged to a computer dating service aggressively hunting.

One hour later I was heading for the door. My tolerance was over. As I was about to step through the exit, a man began talking to me. He said that we had met before. The line did not impress me. When he reminisced about the comedian joking about us, I realized that it was Gabriel. Once again we conversed for a long time, and once again he asked for my phone number. I would have wagered six months' pay that he wouldn't contact me. The next day he called.

Gabriel told me that he had really liked me at our first meeting but was not willing to date someone with children. Three desperate years later, he broke his rule. We dated every weekend for six months. We went to restaurants, movies, plays, street fairs, and tennis matches.

At first I wasn't sure if Gabriel would be around for the long term. I kept waiting to find out what was the matter with him. He was a forty-five-year-old bachelor. Only one prior relationship had lasted for more than a year. I thought maybe that his training to become a physician had hampered his social life. Gabriel explained that he just never met the "right one."

Gabriel was bright, funny, handsome, and a good guy. He was also grateful he had met me. Each night, for over twenty years, he had prayed to God for a wife and future offspring. Then he was presented with me and instant children.

My prior husband was a romantic French Canadian named Pierre. However, subsequently he began romancing other women. Instead of providing us with a third child, he impregnated one of his paramours—a married woman he first contacted on the internet. Now it was a pleasure to have a man who prayed for only one wife and one family.

Following our six months of dating, Gabriel invited me to fly with him to Curaçao over Christmas vacation. My daughters, Elizabeth and Lisette, were with their father for the holidays. When we arrived at the hotel, Gabriel immediately placed a small box in the safe. I thought: engagement ring! Each evening I wore a fancy dress to dinner and waited for Gabriel to "pop the question." Every night I retired to bed without any questions asked.

Our last day in Curaçao, I wore shorts and a T-shirt. We visited the oldest synagogue in the Americas. It was an imposing Sephardic sanctuary. There was a pulpit in the center of the room, high ceilings, and a sand-covered floor. Gabriel went down on his knees in front of the ark where the Torah scrolls are kept, pulled out the little box, and asked me to marry him. I agreed to become his wife, and my answer echoed throughout the temple. Gabriel's timing was perfect. Five minutes later the first camera-wielding mob arrived right off the cruise ship.

Gabriel wanted a "real" wedding with all of the trappings. Since it was his first marriage, it wouldn't have been fair of me to insist on a justice of the peace, two-piece suit, and quiet luncheon second-marriage type of affair. I decided to have the dream wedding that I didn't have the first time. I located a turn-of-the-century wedding gown of handmade Irish lace with a pattern of birds and flowers. We had an outdoor ceremony on the back lawn of an early 1900s mansion. Elizabeth and Lisette marched down first in Elizabethan-style dresses and gracefully tossed roses out of wicker baskets. I felt like a character out of an Edith Wharton novel.

The weather was a ninety-nine-degree heat wave. The rabbi spoke about our having "sunny days" ahead, the "heat" of our love, and the "warmth" of our support. As soon as the ceremony ended, everyone ran inside to the air-conditioning of the mansion turned catering hall.

Later, Gabriel's two best men held up their glasses and congratulated a member of their longstanding singles group for finally getting married. My daughters returned from the mansion's bowling alley just in time to hear the end of the toast. Elizabeth, my oldest daughter, announced that she wanted to make a toast too. She held up a glass of Coke and said, "I want to say that I know we will become a happy family. Ever since five years ago when I 'lost' my father I was wishing for a new one. Now he's here. I know he'll be a great dad. My life is just beginning." All of the women were drying their eyes with their cocktail napkins.

A few days after the wedding, Elizabeth and Lisette left for a month of sleep-away camp. Gabriel and I departed on a two-week honeymoon. We went to a romantic town called Eze in the south of France. Our hotel was a medieval structure built into the side of a cliff;

the outdoor restaurant posted a warning not to drop anything, because it could not be retrieved from the bottom of the precipice. Fortunately neither of us had a fear of heights.

Gabriel and I spent the last two weeks moving into our new home. We enjoyed our month of marriage with just the two of us, and then we became a "readymade" family when the children returned from camp.

I was lucky to marry Gabriel. Now I also would be successful with creating a baby. The doctor was definitely wrong. No amount of scientific advances could obliterate the magical element of procreation. Even in ancient times the women knew that the spark of life must be stoked to ignite in their wombs. The Egyptians and Romans left offerings for their fertility goddesses. Modern-day technology might not guarantee my baby. But luck would.

The next step was my hospital orientation. I expected a freshman orientation like one at college. The women would have a chance to bond. We would embark on our baby journey together. At graduation, instead of a diploma, we would all be handed a baby.

The orientation office looked like a lawyer's conference room. There was a long, rectangular mahogany table with matching wood chairs, paneled wood walls, and a smiling nurse standing at the end of the table. The participants were all couples except me. Once again, my husband couldn't leave work. We all sat down and waited to get oriented.

This was not an introduction to freshman fertility life at the hospital. We were not introduced to each other. Our nurse lecturer wore a lab coat and nametag. We rapidly were immersed in IVF 101.

"We will see who makes it into the upcoming IVF trial. You won't all make it. It depends on the start of your next period. Plus naturally we have shut-down times like Christmas and part of the summer."

Now that I had made it to this meeting because of my acceptable hormone levels, I did not want to be excluded from the trial. I wanted to start right away. Hopefully my period would comply.

The nurse proceeded to educate us about the protocol.

"When you get your natural period you must test for ovulation. Eight to ten days after the home ovulation test registers positive, you start your Lupron shots. That will give you a Lupron period. The

Lupron period is very special. It's a controlled period that suppresses your hormones."

I felt as if I was back in ninth-grade health class, learning about menstruation and childbirth all over again. In that class, after watching a film of a woman screaming in agony as she pushed out her infant, I had vowed never to have a baby. In this one I was trying my hardest to become pregnant.

The nurse joyously continued.

"Three days after your Lupron period, you start hormones. But we have a busy hospital schedule. We must coordinate many women. Don't be impatient. A day-three period might be day seven. It all depends when you fit in. When you do come in for your day three start, be sure to sign in on the pink sheet. If you sign in on the white sheet we might forget to call you."

This was becoming confusing: now I had to remember the color of the paper and the correct start date. Then the nurse began talking about injections.

"All of you have a shot assignment in your packet. It lists your prescribed hormones. These will be administered either in the abdomen, which we call subcutaneous, or in your buttocks—intramuscular."

I searched through my packet to find my hormones. I was assigned Gonal F for my stomach and Pergonol for my rear. In addition I still would be getting Lupron in the stomach.

I hated shots. I was even afraid of the fingerprick to test my blood sugar levels. When I was little, I had prepared myself for my pediatric injections by pretending that I was a soldier in a war. Soon every day I would have to conjure up battlefield acts of heroics as Gabriel stabbed me with the needle. I did not yet know that I would be imagining airplane runways or that Gabriel would try to comfort me with his buzzing bees.

The nurse went on with her lecture.

"Once you start your additional hormones, you'll be in regularly for hospital visits. You must arrive no later than eight-forty-five in the morning. Your blood will be monitored to determine if your medication doses must be changed. Your follicle size and production level will be followed by sonograms. Every afternoon we'll call you with the level of hormones to take that evening."

I kept focusing on the part about getting to the hospital by 8:45. Now that was going to be a problem! It meant getting up before dawn each morning to catch a train, having blood drawn, and rushing to work on no sleep. When I was sleep-deprived, I couldn't think straight. As a psychologist with a private practice, it was imperative for me to concentrate on what my patients were saying. I hoped I wouldn't become so disoriented that I'd mix up my patients.

"I don't want to alarm all of you, but we must discuss the pitfalls," continued our nurse.

"You can go into hyperstimulation. That's when you make too many follicles and your hormone levels skyrocket too quickly. This can result in a twisted ovary, blood clots, and even death. Some of you might not even respond to the medication. You also could have a dominant follicle, which would grow before all the others and cause the others to stop developing. Then you would have only one good egg left for IVF. One is not enough. Unfortunately, you then would be eliminated from the trial."

Just as I was beginning to feel like a first-year medical student who "caught" every disease that was studied, the nurse proclaimed enthusiastically, "Now it's time to learn all the new terminology. First of all, when your eggs are ready to come out they will be *harvested.*" The nurse put a lot of emphasis on our new word. "This will be the day of your egg *retrieval.* The egg will be retrieved from the follicle that contains it. Each egg will need to be fertilized by the sperm. You might need the procedure called ICSI—intracytoplasmic sperm injections. ICSI is when the sperm is directly injected into the egg. Any questions yet?"

I did not ask any questions, even though I found the information confusing. No one else asked any questions either. They were probably just as quietly lost as I was. The nurse proceeded, "The fertilized eggs will be placed back into the uterus on either day three or day five. A day-five transfer is at the blastocyst stage. There's more embryonic development at that point and therefore an increased rate of a successful pregnancy—in fact there could be a much higher rate of implantation than with a day-three transfer. However, not everyone can wait until day five because the embryo might stop developing since it's still outside of the womb. Then there would be nothing at all to transfer."

Another booby trap. If they waited until the fifth day my baby might die in the test tube, but if they transferred the baby into my womb at day three it had less chance of sticking. I didn't want to hear about possible complications. Better the Scarlett O'Hara approach of "Tomorrow is another day" without worrying whether I reached three or five tomorrows.

The nurse continued. "The embryologist may elect to utilize *assisted hatching*. Assisted hatching is when the shell of the egg is scraped in one corner in order to help with attachment to the wall of the uterus. How many eggs are placed will depend on the age of the patient. Younger women have a greater chance of multiple births and we want to reduce the chances of multiple births. Therefore, we will place fewer eggs. In contrast, the egg quality of older women is not as good so they are unlikely to have multiple births. We can comfortably transfer five or six eggs without worrying about a lot of resulting children."

Finally there was a question: a heavyset man began to wave his arm wildly.

"I need your help. I want to make sure my wife has at least two babies. Four or five would be preferable. I want her to have them all at once. Then she can go back to work, and I'll stay home with the babies," explained the man.

"We don't want multiple births. Your wife would be placed on bed rest and the babies could have complications."

"I never said I wanted all of those babies," chimed in his wife, a tiny, slender woman who was about a foot shorter than her husband and two hundred pounds lighter.

The nurse said, "I can talk with you both about all of this later."

Soon afterward someone else's husband, with slicked-back hair and an expensive suit, began questioning the nurse. He argued about the hospital's probability statistics and thought the success rates were inflated. I was positive he was a lawyer.

Finally the nurse shook him off by stating, "It's time for our slide show." Now I watched photos of an egg being injected with a sperm via ICSI, an egg being hatched, and a day-three and a day-five embryo that were each ready for transfer.

The lights went back on. It was time for our lesson on preparing the vials of hormones. We were each provided with a vial filled with liquid, a hypodermic needle, and bottles of powder. First we learned how to twist the glass vial so it would break. Mine wasn't opening, and I was tempted to tap it open like an egg. However, with a little help it worked. Next we took our needles and practiced drawing liquid into them. We had to measure the correct cubic centimeters of liquid and place the liquid into the jars with powder that represented our hormone medication. The experience reminded me of eighth-grade chemistry class.

"Now, this will be fun!" exclaimed the nurse. She was holding the torso of a mannequin. "For the finale of our class you get to practice giving injections into the butt of the mannequin." The first husband to practice jammed the needle right into the center of one of the mannequin's butt cheeks. "Your wife would be in a lot of pain if you administered the injection that way," the nurse said. Patiently, she told us to first push some liquid out of the needle to avoid air bubbles, to place the needle in an outer quadrant of the buttocks to avoid nerve endings, to enter via a muscle, and then to smoothly and gracefully place the needle. "Afterward, to reduce pain, the area should be massaged and hot compresses placed on the buttocks," advised the nurse. We all got a few turns wielding our needles.

Last came the financial section. The cost of each trial was about ten thousand dollars, not including the hormones (which could be more than five thousand dollars), or any additional recommended procedures such as ICSI or hatching. Payment in full would be due at the start of the trial. If you were one of the ones dropped from the trial for whatever reason, you would receive a refund minus whatever procedures had already been implemented. All payments must be made in full unless you participated with the one insurance company the hospital accepted.

By the completion of the orientation, I felt overwhelmed and dazed rather than enlightened. The clearest communication was how much money I would owe the hospital. Yet I still wanted to embark on my IVF journey, despite the obstacles, because my baby beckoned at the end.

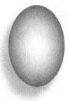

The Pink Sheet

The requisite three days from the start of my Lupron period, I was back in the hospital to begin my trial and to undergo my first blood test. I remembered to sign my name on the pink sheet. Now I was official. The receptionist sat behind a big mahogany counter covered with sign-in sheets. I turned around to look for a chair, but there were no seats! Over a hundred people were in the waiting room.

Finally someone was called, and I found a seat. I was surprised at the number of women with infertility problems. Some women in the waiting room were my contemporaries. They wore impeccable business suits, the perfect amount of make-up, and becoming hairstyles. I was sure that they had important corporate careers and had delayed motherhood too long. Since I'd successfully conceived and delivered two children I thought that I was in a separate category, that I had a leg up on these "virgin pregnancy" women. Then there were the very young women in their twenties. A number were Orthodox Jews wearing wigs and accompanied by husbands with beards, long sideburns, and yarmulkes. The twenty-year-olds must have severe fertility problems to be here at their age. I was positive that I was different from everyone else and destined to succeed.

Determined to relax, I pulled out my book about King Henry VIII and his wives. I was reading about Anne Boleyn. She was waiting to provide Henry VIII with a son. Henry had cast off his devoted wife of more than twenty years and changed the religion of the land in order to marry her, even though Anne was already in her thirties and not that nubile either. Anne's older sister Mary Boleyn had been one of Henry's prior lovers. Anne not only had to compete with her sister, but she also had to justify the extreme actions taken by Henry to wed her. Henry and Anne were confidently printing all the announcements ahead of time with the word "prince." The "prince" announcements had to be changed when Anne gave birth to the future Elizabeth I. Her fertility attempt was a success, but she still failed the more stringent royal requirement of a male heir. Only centuries later would genetics vindicate her and reveal that it was the "Y" chromosome of the male that determined the sex and that it was the "fault" of Henry that she bore him a son.

Josephine Bonaparte also was in my thoughts. I'd just finished reading a biography of her for my book club. She too tried to create a baby to continue an empire. Although she had two children from a previous marriage, she was unable to provide Napoleon a child. Like me, her two children were already older when she tried for a third. Josephine was in her thirties, but she entered into early menopause. The cause was thought to be from the trauma of being locked in the Bastille waiting to be guillotined. Josephine endured numerous invasive and painful "treatments" in the hopes of regaining her menstrual flow. Her treatments included leeches, laxatives, and dousings in spring water. Napoleon ultimately discarded Josephine in order to conceive a son with Princess Marie-Louise of Austria.

I did not feel in danger of being beheaded like Anne Boleyn or being cast off like Josephine Bonaparte for a younger, more fertile wife. My husband felt lucky to be married. But I knew that he too wanted a male.

My husband also had a famous bloodline to uphold. Gabriel was the eighth-generation descendant in an unbroken male line. The line went back to Lithuania. The bearded man who began the lineage was a renowned sage, a brilliant philosopher who led his people. His name was Elijah ben Solomon, and he was known as the Vilna Gaon (the genius of Vilna). He was one of the most important religious scholars of the time, and Gabriel grew up with this family legend. The man also was a child prodigy who at age ten outstripped and fired his tutors. He could be looked up in the *Encyclopedia Britannica*. There was even a museum exhibit about him. The exhibit included a family tree. My husband and his father were on the tree. Also on the tree was Mr. Spock, the Vulcan from the original *Star Trek* series. Apparently Leonard Nimoy was a descendant as well.

The sage was so learned that he could not take time away from his studying of the Talmud. He decided to stop talking to his wife and children. In contrast to his ancestor, Gabriel was putting family first. He would need to focus on me and on our fertility in order to continue the unbroken lineage.

Gabriel also had parents who hoped to be expectant grandparents. They had been patiently waiting almost thirty years. Gabriel's father was now ninety-four and his mother was ninety. They were exuberant when their only child married at age forty-six. In fact, Gabriel was just following in their footsteps. His parents had married at ages forty-three and thirty-nine. His mother conceived Gabriel at age forty-two after numerous miscarriages from a previously undiagnosed polyp.

Gabriel joked that his parents were a "two-walker household." His father went to dialysis three times a week and belted "Hava Nagila" as he pushed his walker to and from the dialysis machine. His father also yelled at his mother, but that was because she could not hear a thing. A bigger hearing aid might have done the trick, but she didn't want to wear the larger, more prominent one.

At our wedding Gabriel's father looked dapper in a tuxedo, and his mother wore a pretty, pink dress. During the outdoor ceremony, they both sported Mexican sombreros to keep the sun off their faces. They also each carried a portable, battery-operated fan in one hand and a water bottle in the other. They already were looking forward to buying new outfits for their grandchild's baby naming ceremony.

Like Gabriel, I also grew up with a family legend, but mine was the story of the orphanage where my father lived as a boy. His parents had been high school sweethearts who ran off to be married against their parents' wishes. My grandfather was a handsome, charismatic ladies' man and my grandmother Lola a sexy, dark-haired beauty who wore low-cut blouses to display her ample cleavage. In later years, my father discovered naked photos that my grandfather had taken of my grandmother with discreetly placed fig leaves.

Shortly after my father turned six, my grandmother decided that she could no longer put up with my grandfather's stream of lovers and delivered my father to an orphanage. Week after week my father sat at a long dining table and ate with his fellow orphans in an Oliver Twist–style setting. Every Sunday he sat on the front steps expectantly waiting for someone to visit. Mostly no one ever did. Once in a while my great-grandmother, a proud German woman who grew up wealthy in a Fifth Avenue townhouse, stopped by to see her grandson. However, she never took him home with her. My father vowed to himself that one day he would show them all and make something of himself.

Eventually, after my grandmother married her second husband, a chicken plucker called "Chickie," she arrived on the scene to reclaim her son. Unfortunately, she had never told her new husband about the existence of her son. Chickie was very unhappy to become a father and never got along with his stepson.

In the end, my father loved his mother for taking him back. In later years, he supported her financially. My father fulfilled his orphanage vow and became a doctor who made life-saving discoveries. My grandmother Lola never changed. When she first welcomed my mother into her house, she greeted her in a black negligée. My grandmother generously supplied me with her choice books, beginning with *Valley of the Dolls*.

The part of the legend that most affected me was my father sitting by himself on the front step of the orphanage waiting for parents who never came. I imagined what it was like to feel abandoned and alone. I myself was a sensitive child who reacted strongly to perceived rejection. As a child, I vowed to have a close-knit family when I grew up and always to be there for my children and for my spouse. Being betrayed by my first husband made it all the more important for everything to go right the second time. I was convinced that a baby of our own would really cement my marriage. This time I would have a family that lasted, where everyone was valued.

I also really wanted this baby. Originally I had wanted to duplicate my family of origin and have only two children. However, like Gabriel with his initial decision not to date a woman with children, I too could change my game plan. Having two girls in diapers did not discourage me from future babies. Elizabeth was great fun as she threw the pillows onto the living room floor and shouted one of her first words. Lisette was an agile monkey who climbed the built-in shelves in the living room as if she were scaling a palm tree and threw down china plates as if discarding banana peels. I relished the uniqueness of each daughter and surprised myself by wanting another child. Now I could enjoy raising another baby. Plus I would be sharing it this time with Gabriel, who was very loving and committed. I was as positive as Anne Boleyn that I would fulfill my own as well as my husband's expectations for a baby.

The woman next to me in the waiting room made eye contact and smiled. "I'm crocheting something. In fact I'm crocheting constantly in order to avoid having a breakdown," she explained frantically.

I told her, "I'm glad that you like crocheting and that it's soothing for you." I returned to reading about the upcoming decapitation of Anne Boleyn.

"Victoria Hopewell!" called the nurse. I followed her into the next room. She walked with the purposeful strut of a model on a runway. There were two rows of cubicles with women lined up in chairs getting their blood drawn. I sat down in my chair to wait for my first IVF trial bloodletting. The woman tied a piece of material across my right arm, told me to grasp a rubber ball, and prepared to draw my blood.

She stuck the needle into my vein. "I don't understand it. The vein looks good but not much blood is coming out. I'll just move the needle around. That's not working, I'll try to press harder and see if we can get that blood coming. Oh, here we go!" I started to feel very lightheaded and my eyes started to close. When I opened my eyes, I saw a group of white lab coats fluttering above me. One of the lab coats came closer and a face appeared. "You just fainted. Why don't you lie down in the back room until you feel better." I hoped that this wasn't indicative of the rest of my blood-drawing sessions!

The next needles were administered at home by my husband. My shots increased. "Bend over, lean forward, put your hands on the bed to steady yourself. Now here comes the buzzing bee. Get ready for the next little sting, just a tiny prick, *now!*" warned my husband. I yelped again. The new position of leaning forward was only a slight improvement over the prior position of lying prone across the bed. The Pergonal subcutaneous, in-the-butt shots were much worse than the

Lupron and Gonal F into the stomach. Every night my children had story time, and I had shot time.

My next trip to the hospital was for blood drawing and for an internal exam. This time I was lucky and found a waiting room seat right away.

"Hi! I'm Brittany," said the woman next to me.

"And I'm Dakota," chimed in the woman to her right.

They proceeded to explain their IVF story to me. Brittany and Dakota were sisters. They were tall, willowy women who resembled Nicole Kidman. Indeed Dakota was an actress in soap operas. Dakota had flown in from Australia to donate her eggs to Brittany, who'd flown in from London. Although she was only thirty-one, Brittany's eggs were not of good quality. Dakota got all the injections, monitoring of her blood levels, and examinations of her follicle production. Brittany accompanied her to all appointments and eventually would receive the eggs harvested from her sister. Dakota told me that she loved her sister and if necessary would fly in again for her egg donation. It was a real testament to sibling love that one sister would fly all those miles to share her eggs with the other; I hoped that Elizabeth and Lisette would be that supportive of each other one day. It also made me feel more confident in the hospital, since Brittany and Dakota had chosen it out of all the fertility programs around the world.

I was glad that the sisters made contact with me. Most people in the waiting room were quiet and uncommunicative. They respected each other's privacy and did not confide in each other. The atmosphere was of oppressive, individual suffering. But once a conversation started with someone, bonding was quick. There was a built-in connection and the possibility of future waiting room meetings.

"Victoria Hopewell!" I went to the cubicle for my blood drawing. It was the same nurse who couldn't get my blood to come out! I had visions of landing on the floor this time. "Don't worry. I'm sure you won't faint," the nurse reassured me. This time she jabbed the needle with one big movement, the blood came out right away, and I didn't faint, but I had a big purple bruise on my arm. "Now go back out and wait to be called for your ultrasound," she instructed.

When I went back out, I looked for the sisters, but they had already been called in. There was a seat in the back, where a group of people, in contrast to the rest of the silent gang, usually sat together talking and laughing loudly. The most outspoken woman from the group, a brunette with a chubby face, introduced herself and the others. She explained that they all met online in an IVF chat room. Her name was Lauren, and she appeared to be the group leader by virtue of her holding the IVF veteran record. This was her eighth attempt. Lauren knew the story of every other group member, information about every IVF doctor at the hospital, questions that we should ask the doctors, and detailed information about each procedure.

When a woman ran out from the room crying, Lauren explained to the rest of us that it was because one of her follicles had become dominant—one of the elimination pitfalls described by the orientation nurse. The doctor had just informed the weeping woman that her trial was aborted, Lauren said—one viable egg was not enough for implantation.

I felt conflicted during these ad hoc connections because I did not tell my newfound friends that I already had two children. I was afraid that if I did tell them, I would be excluded from the camaraderie of the mutual baby quest.

My name was called again, and I went in for my sonogram appointment. The nurse had me put my feet in the stirrups and wait for the doctor. He said hello, remained nameless, and got right to business. The sonogram displayed the contents of my right ovary and then my left. The exact measurements of each follicle were diligently recorded. Unfortunately, the sonogram also displayed a large cyst. The doctor explained that cyst development was normal at ovulation. However, for IVF to be successful it was imperative that there be no cyst. If it didn't disappear over the next four or five days, from my hormone medication, then I would be scheduled for immediate cyst aspiration.

A few days later, I knew that I would have to undergo this "spring cleaning," because the cyst did not disappear. Since I required surgery, I decided that it was time to inform my daughters about IVF and our baby quest. Already I was disappearing each morning, returning with bandages from the blood drawings. Elizabeth and Lisette needed to know something. I was not sure how they would react to a new sibling. We were not the Brady Bunch but the children had adjusted well and even called their stepfather "Dad." Now our new family would have to survive the shake-up of a baby.

Gabriel and I sat the girls down in the dining room. We began our baby discussion.

"We have something to tell you girls. Your father and I are planning to have a baby."

"I never got to experience a baby because I met your mother when you were already older," added Gabriel.

"I am going to get some help becoming pregnant from a hospital because I'm older now. The hospital has a program to help people. They will take my eggs out and put the best ones back," I explained.

"That's not all they do! I know all about it already," said Elizabeth.

I asked, "From health class?"

She said, "No, from religious school from my ethics class."

"I want you girls to know that we'll always love you. We just want to have one child together," I said.

"I don't want a baby!" exclaimed Lisette.

"Mom has no chance anyway at her age," said Elizabeth. "What about our puppy? You promised us if we ever moved out of our apartment and back into a house we'd get a puppy."

"I want a puppy too!" added Lisette.

"Well, we can have a puppy and a baby," I said.

I was positive that the children would ensure that we got the puppy. It would be up to the hospital to enable Gabriel and me to get the baby.

"If you do get a baby I only want a girl. Then I'll be the one to pick out its clothes. We'll wear the same jeans and shirts," said Lisette.

"You can be the baby's personal shopper," I said.

I would have preferred if the girls were excited about a new baby. Once I became pregnant they'd have more time to adjust to the idea. Then maybe they'd become more accepting of their new sibling.

As soon as our conversation ended, Elizabeth was on the phone telling her friends that her mother's eggs were being removed and returned to make a baby. I was sure all of her friends' brothers, sisters, mothers, and fathers also heard about my eggs as well.

I also decided to share with my parents that we would be having a baby. I expected them to be proud, happy grandparents. I wouldn't get too detailed about IVF. My mother was a product of the 1950s, and we had never even discussed the "normal" means of procreation. She often repeated the story of how she had met my father on a cruise for college students. My mother explained that it was a wild boat, that she encountered my father the first day, but that he had disappeared until the last day of the trip, presumably to be with "the other type of girls." Then when the cruise was over, he asked for my mother's number. They began dating and my mother married him during spring break of her senior year at Wellesley. She was able to remain in the dormitory, while my father finished his last year of medical school in New York, because she signed an agreement not to reveal the dark secrets of married life to the still pure Wellesley virgins. The only sexual thing that my mother ever said to me was imparted right before I left for college, when she told me, "Once it's broken, it's broken."

I waited for my father's History Channel program on ancient Rome to finish before I broke the news. "Mom and Dad, you're going to be grandparents again. Soon there'll be a new baby. Gabriel and I haven't been able to get pregnant on our own so we're going to a doctor for help. I'll be taking hormones."

"Hormones? Hormones! That'll give you cancer. My mother died of a melanoma. Why would you take hormones?" my mother cried.

"So that I can get pregnant."

"Victoria, you're too old for that. Just think of the damage you'll cause your body by carrying a baby to term and then giving birth. Afterward you'll need a wheelchair, possibly for life."

"I'll be okay."

"Plus at your age the baby will probably have Downs Syndrome."

"Mom, it should be fine."

"Victoria, I think this is a very bad idea."

"Don't you want a grandchild?"

"I already have four—your two and your brother's two, and I'm only concerned about your health."

"Well, I'm going to do it anyway."

My father chimed in. "Victoria, don't you think you're too old to be a parent again?"

"No. I want to have a baby with Gabriel."

"You have to really think about what it means to start all over again with an infant. You'll be changing diapers, losing sleep, and spending the next eighteen years raising a child again. You'll be stuck."

"I don't mind."

"Well, it's your life."

My parents weren't the proud grandparents that I had hoped. I knew that my father would be more matter-of-fact than my mother. In the end he had always told me to make my own decisions. Still I would have liked it if he could see some joy for Gabriel and me in starting a family of our own. I wouldn't tell them about my cyst operation in a week; that would really put them over the edge—especially my mother.

When I arrived a week later for my cyst aspiration, the receptionist immediately announced, "Boy, you're brave!" Her large, rhinestone barrette sparkled under the bright ceiling lights.

"What do you mean?"

"It's great that you don't want any anesthesia for your procedure. There are some people who make that choice."

"I didn't request 'no anesthesia.' I don't want to have any pain. I'm all for killing the pain. You'd better tell someone right away that I definitely did not request to have nothing."

"Don't worry, just tell the doctor," soothed the receptionist.

As soon as the doctor arrived, I told him that I didn't want to feel anything, that I wanted anesthesia or a "local." He flashed me a big smile. "It's not necessary," he said. "I'll be real quick. I'll just insert the needle into the vagina, look at the ultrasound for guidance, and aspirate the cyst." I started shaking at the thought of a big needle entering me. The doctor said, "I'm doing it right now." I felt the needle stab me, and the pain was immediate. Still, the terror beforehand was worse than the actual impact of the needle. The doctor was pleased because the procedure was a success, and I would not have to recover from anesthesia.

I waited for my husband to pick me up from the cyst aspiration. Everyone else had left except for the receptionist. I told her that I'd be back soon for the egg retrieval. The receptionist confided that when she began this job, she thought that it would be a happy scenario. She envisioned numerous new mothers coming back to visit her with their newborn babies. In fact she saw most people again when they returned as "repeaters." I told her, "Well, hopefully you won't see me again after the trial unless it's with my baby!" Her words did not discourage me. I still felt that my luck would hold and that I'd be one of the few destined to return with an infant in my arms.

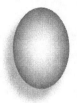

Halfway Road to Pregnancy

My eggs were finally ready to be harvested and retrieved. The hCG (human chorionic gonadotropin) shot had to be given at exactly midnight so that my follicles would release my eggs thirty-four to thirty-six hours later. The doctors wanted everything coordinated for my assigned morning egg retrieval time.

The night of the shot, I was invited to my friend's anniversary party. It was a holiday weekend. There was a chance that I wouldn't be back by twelve if there was traffic. Therefore, I had to be prepared. The hCG, syringe, alcohol swabs, and disposal waste case were all packed. If necessary we'd pull to the side of the highway, I'd lift my cocktail dress, and expose my backside to the people driving by while I waited for the buzzing bee to land. Luckily we made it back before midnight.

I arrived early in the morning for my egg harvesting. I was handed a brown paper shopping bag and told to go change. The changing room was similar to one at our community pool, with a wooden bench and a clothing hook on the door. My new outfit consisted of slippers, drawstring cloth pants, a wraparound sleeveless shirt with ties, a robe, and a blue cloth shower cap.

The husbands were being called one by one for their sperm deposits. My husband was called next. Gabriel went into a room with a comfortable reclining chair. There was a large supply of magazines with naked women, a few magazines of naked men, and a television hooked up to a VCR with an X-rated video lying next to it: a hospital version of a Times Square peep show—with private room so husbands could participate fully in the excitement of the spectacle. Earlier, the receptionist had announced that if any man experienced difficulty, his wife could be called in to assist. My husband did not experience any difficulty. He placed the filled cup into a hole in the wall, closed the little sliding door, and rang the bell to announce that his deposit was ready for pickup. At least one of us was having fun.

When Gabriel returned, we were prepared to wait a while but it turned out that I was in the first group called. The women were divided into groups of three. Lauren was in my group, as well as a younger woman in her twenties named Courtney. Courtney had angled brown hair with the shortest pieces falling into her eyes.

The three of us followed the nurse to a tiny waiting area. Lauren started to tell me what to expect. I would receive anesthesia via intravenous and would be "out" for about twenty-five minutes. When I woke up I would find out how many eggs were removed.

Lauren went first. Courtney and I started talking. Courtney was only twenty-six, but she and her husband weren't able to get pregnant on their own. This was her first IVF attempt, but she had gone through multiple trials of artificial insemination. All of a sudden I saw Lauren being wheeled by. She was lying unconscious on the gurney wearing the operating outfit with the matching blue cap. Courtney was called next. I tried to read the celebrity magazine on the table and get absorbed in who was seeing whom. My concentration was broken when I saw Courtney being wheeled back from the operating room. Next it was my turn. I wondered if the following group of three would see my unconscious body being wheeled by—not a relaxing preparation for surgery.

Soon I was back in the same room where my cyst had been aspirated. There were bright lights shining on me as I lay across the operating table. At least this time anesthesia was a definite. I was hooked up intravenously, just as Lauren told me. A trail of tubes protruded from my hand. I did not go under right away, however, but watched while the doctor and nurse prepared their utensils. I'd better go under real soon, I thought, because I did not want to be awake for the birth of my eggs.

When I woke up I was on the bed with curtains pulled all around me in the communal post-operation room. The nurse brought in my husband. She shared the good news that I was the producer of seventeen eggs. My husband and I were still in the running!

The side curtain started to move. Lauren's husband was pulling the curtain, and there was Lauren lying on the adjacent recovery bed.

"I just wanted to see how you did," she said.

"I had seventeen eggs."

"That's great!" she exclaimed. "I set my record with twenty-five eggs!"

We exchanged phone numbers.

The next afternoon we would find out how many eggs had been successfully fertilized. The nurse would tell me. Since a sperm was inserted into each egg, I was sure all seventeen would be fertilized. However, when the nurse called me she said about half of my eggs were fertilized—nine. Well, nine was still great. I should even have eggs left over to freeze for the future!

The next day the nurse would call to say whether my eggs would be returned at day three or day five. I feared the worst, and sure enough my eggs were a day-three transfer. The nurse tried to comfort me by saying that most people were a day-three transfer because it was too risky to wait for day five and possibly lose all the eggs.

When I returned for my egg transfer, Lauren was in the waiting area again. She told me every one of her eggs had been fertilized. In order to increase her chances, she had instructed the doctor to place the eggs back using a sonogram and to "hatch" every one so that they would adhere better. She wanted as many eggs placed back as possible. Lauren's doctor had already called her a number of times and told her the egg quality was good. I hadn't heard from my doctor since our initial meeting. Lauren asked me to pray for her because this was her last chance: every one of her credit cards was "maxed out."

The same order was observed for us three women. Lauren's eggs were put back first. Courtney was there again, and we started to talk. She had produced thirty-one eggs! I guess being in your twenties did make a big difference. She went in next, and I wished her good luck.

Finally it was my turn. I had to sign a paper stating that I was who I claimed to be. I suppose they didn't want the wrong person getting my eggs. The embryologist arrived and with an air of great importance hand-delivered my set of fertilized eggs from the lab. Above me, a screen displayed a picture of each of my viable fertilized eggs. At this point there were only five. The other four had "demonstrated abnormal fertilization." No more frozen eggs. It was these five. Three embryos had divided eight times and two had divided six times. The doctor said eight and six were good numbers. It was like a Las Vegas craps table.

Thanks to Lauren's information, I asked the doctor whether he would guide my eggs back into place with the use of a sonogram. "No," he said. He was of the old school and could slide my eggs back into the uterus without it. He was like an experienced safe cracker; he said he had a natural feel for the combination. Then I asked if my eggs were "hatched." He said neither the embryologist or my doctor had recommended it. The doctor put my eggs back successfully, then double-checked that they were in the right location without spilling any on the floor.

My souvenir was a color picture of the five eggs. I could differentiate those with six divisions from the eight-division ones. There also was a score card. It delineated the history of all seventeen. From the eight eggs that didn't fertilize, three were "immature," two "appeared degenerative," two had "morphology unsuitable for transfer," and one "appeared healthy and did not become fertilized." Each non-viable egg was a personal failure. About 50 percent of my total production was deformed. I was so identified with my eggs that it was as if something was the matter with me too. I wondered if I was going to have a baby or if I just was going to have a picture of five fertilized eggs and a score card to put in my baby album.

Next I was wheeled back into the recovery room with its large collection of beds with curtains around them. There was no anesthesia, so I was totally awake. The nurse told me to rest for a half hour before going home.

Lauren screamed out, "Victoria! How did it go?"

It turned out that she was next to me again.

"I had five eggs put back," I answered.

Lauren told me that she had eight eggs returned. Her eggs all had divided to stage ten or twelve. She said she'd call the next day.

Lauren called the next morning. She told me that she was staying in bed with her legs up to enhance egg implantation. Her mother was coming for a week to help so that she could remain in bed and increase her chances.

I confided that I had accidentally moved a box. There was no heavy lifting allowed, and I was worried that maybe I knocked out an egg from the womb. Lauren told me that the eggs probably didn't implant yet. She said wait to feel a marked cramp—that would tell me an egg had implanted. She explained that every time that she had become pregnant from a trial (although no baby of hers had ever gone to term), she always felt this sharp pain. I told her I'd wait for the pain. I was going back to work the next day, but for today I was in bed—but without my legs in the air.

Later that evening I actually did feel a sharp pain! I was ecstatic that I might be pregnant. I began to watch for signs of nausea because I had strong morning sickness while pregnant with my daughters.

Brittany, the sister who received the eggs from Dakota, called me. We had met one more time while getting blood drawn and exchanged numbers. She was upset because Dakota had made only three eggs and only one fertilized. However, it was of good quality and the egg had been transferred back. Her doctor informed her that the chances were about 20 percent now that only one egg was transferred.

The phone rang. It was Lauren. She was very "bummed out." This time she hadn't felt "the cramp," and she didn't feel the same as the other times when she was pregnant. I said that doesn't mean anything and that this pregnancy could be different. Lauren told me how to determine ahead of time if I was pregnant. It all depended on the estradiol and progesterone hormone levels. The hospital had taken them for research purposes only, but Lauren informed me that a high estradiol level probably meant pregnant and that if two days later it was even higher I was most definitely pregnant. Otherwise I probably was not. I told her I'd call the hospital and compare results with her.

Lauren called, ecstatic. Her first estradiol level was 500! She might be pregnant. One person from her IVF chat room group had an estradiol of 300, and she was pregnant. The one with an estradiol of 60 was not pregnant. I told her that my estradiol was less than 32—it didn't sound promising.

After speaking with Lauren, I called the IVF nurse and asked about my estradiol.

She said, "Estradiol is not always a good predictor."

"Can you tell anything from the estradiol level?" I asked.

"All I can say is that the estradiol levels should be increasing over time."

I hoped mine would be higher next time.

But my estradiol went down to less than 20. I was definitely not pregnant. Plus I did the "three days in advance of your missed period" home pregnancy test, and it did not show the necessary second pink line. I'd even looked under a magnifying glass, but there was only one pink line to be seen.

Lauren called again. Her estradiol had gone from 500 to 1,000! Lauren was sure she was pregnant and in fact carrying more than one child. Now I was the one who was not at all encouraged.

Brittany called me too. I told her the estradiol trick. She called the nurse to find out her two levels. Hers were also abysmally low.

It was very difficult waiting. As much as I wished that my family could be united before the birth of a baby, the four of us were still adjusting to living together as a family. Tensions remained, mostly between Gabriel and Lisette. This was consistent with my younger daughter's first reactions to Gabriel.

I had waited four months before introducing him to the children. They had never been introduced to any other men I dated. However, Gabriel seemed promising. I carefully orchestrated the initial encounter to take place at an amusement park. That way, I figured, the girls would be on their best behavior. They would be so excited to go on the rides that there would be no blowout fights between them.

Elizabeth, almost age eleven, was charming. She greeted Gabriel with a big smile and chatted as adeptly as any high-society hostess. She squealed with delight when Gabriel shot basketballs into hoops and won her a plush chimpanzee. Elizabeth already knew that Gabriel was her ticket out.

Elizabeth had been affected the most by the divorce. While I was still with her father, she overheard our fights and reprimanded her dad by saying, "Daddy, you shouldn't have a girlfriend." When Pierre and I had the family divorce discussion in front of the fireplace in the living room, we told Elizabeth and Lisette that Pierre wanted to live alone (we left out the part about his going on an out-of-state sabbatical to be with his married lover). Elizabeth shrieked, "No, Daddy, please don't go, don't go, don't do this!"

Then we had to sell our home. The new owners insisted on immediate occupancy. Elizabeth, Lisette, and I moved into one room at our kind elderly neighbor's home so that Elizabeth could finish first grade. We could look out the window of our room and view our former yard with the children's swing set. Elizabeth began running into the woods crying. Our eighty-year-old landlady and I would go looking for her.

When we moved that fall to the town where I grew up, Elizabeth started second grade at her new school. Her classmates thought that she was mute. When she finally began to speak, she only talked about her old school. For back-to-school night, Elizabeth hung up a composition about how her father left the family. Once Elizabeth got a best friend, everything changed. She blossomed socially and academically and was placed in the gifted program at school.

We had moved into an apartment a few blocks from the other side of the railroad tracks. The rest of the community resided in fancy houses. When I was shown our apartment, I kept looking for the second bedroom. The realtor explained that it was a "Junior Four." I could sleep in the dining room with the closing glass doors, and the girls could sleep in the bedroom. The place was already at the top end of my budget so I leased it anyway.

Later the living conditions became even more crowded. I started with one psychology job connected to a school. The school gave me the same hours and vacations as Elizabeth and Lisette's. However, in order to afford our Junior Four, I needed to see private patients at night. There was a babysitter to put the children on the school bus, another to take them off the bus, and a third nighttime sitter. If one sitter canceled it had a domino effect and my whole day of work collapsed. Therefore, I went "live in" and hired a nanny. Now there was my bed in the dining room, the girls in the bedroom, and the nanny in the living room. We took turns dining in our two-person eat-in kitchen. Elizabeth was very nice to Gabriel the entire five hours at the amusement park. She saw visions of a house, her own room, and a built-in father.

Lisette, however, who was eight, clutched my hand. After Gabriel accompanied her on one ride at the amusement park, she insisted that the same ride at camp was much better. When Gabriel took my hand, Lisette immediately squeezed between us and grabbed both my hands. Lisette had nothing personal against Gabriel. She just wanted her mother to herself. Also, Lisette had not been as affected by the divorce. She was four at the time and did not understand much. She thought that her father was on an extended business trip. She did not feel hurt and wasn't searching for a replacement father.

Once we were married eight months later, Elizabeth was grateful to Gabriel for the house and the chance to start again with an intact family. Lisette liked Gabriel but still did not want to share her mommy.

Gabriel also needed to adjust. Gabriel had lived alone since high school except for one college roommate in his freshman year. During more than twenty-five years of bachelorhood, he had developed his own way of doing things. He was very neat and organized and knew the correct place for each of his belongings. The children and I were slobs. The children used his towel and toothbrush. They removed the scissors and tape from his drawer and did not return them.

These events were catastrophic for Gabriel, and his mode of survival was to take over the room in the basement. It had white concrete walls and floors, a tiny aboveground window and a real door that closed. His bed, desk, and bookshelf from his previous apartment were all arranged as if he'd never left. Whenever we drove him crazy, Gabriel escaped to his "bachelor pad."

Gabriel was relieved not to attend any more singles events. He had been part of a group of single men and women who had known each other since their twenties and who now were all approaching or in their fifties. They spent many summers together enjoying time-shares in the Hamptons. During the year, they met in New York on Friday nights to attend the plays of the Roundabout Theater group. For winter vacations, the men frequented Club Med. Once we were married, I asked Gabriel to renew his Roundabout subscription so that we could spend time with his friends and enjoy the performances. We were the only couple. In almost thirty years, Gabriel was the sole member of the group who managed to get married.

Gabriel frequently told me how lucky he was to find me. Gabriel maintained faith that he would find his bride, but after so many years there had been doubts. I let him know how happy I was to have married him. Sometimes at night, in bed, I'd ask him if he would have liked me if we'd met in college or when he was in medical school. He assured me that he would have. I wanted to know that Gabriel and I were meant to be together and that he would have wanted me even when he was younger and less desperate.

Gabriel was eager to become the girls' stepfather. He bought a book and audiotape on becoming a parent. Gabriel hoped to impart some of his own values and his love of Judaism. He knew that Pierre still saw the girls occasionally but thought that there was room for both fathers. When the girls returned from a weekend with Pierre, Gabriel went from being "Dad" to "Gabriel." Since my remarriage, after each school vacation visit Pierre supplied the girls with a framed photo of himself. Whenever I straightened their bedrooms, I inadvertently knocked over a few Pierres.

I decided to contact my sleep-away camp friend Star during this pregnancy waiting period. We had known each other since we were fifteen. I met her when she was sitting under a tree reading a book about Bob Dylan. Once camp ended, our parents used to drive us to sleep over at each other's houses. I felt like a wide-eyed country bumpkin of the suburbs, going to stay at my friend's city home in Brooklyn. Star, who had natural Shirley Temple curls, showed me around Manhattan, and we stood on the twofer line to buy half-price tickets to a Broadway show. We had been each other's confidantes for over twenty-five years.

Star had endometriosis. She had tried for years to get pregnant with artificial insemination, but nothing worked. Star had shown me an adoption book that she and her husband had prepared. There were smiling pictures of the two of them and welcoming words about how much they wanted a child. No one had selected them yet.

While on the adoption wait list, Star also tried one IVF cycle. Although she produced nine eggs, none of them fertilized. She was the only patient with no embryos. After her trial, a new doctor became head of the IVF program. He reviewed her chart and determined that the eggs had been harvested too early. Star tried a second IVF trial, and this time the eggs were kept in her follicles longer. At age thirty-nine, Star was successful and nine months later gave birth to her daughter, Jewel.

I saw Star and her husband, Jay, as my IVF gurus. They knew about it from personal experience, support groups, and professionally. Star also was very active with RESOLVE: The National Infertility Association. She talked to other couples who were striving to have babies. Her husband was a physician's assistant for a doctor who dealt with infertility issues. Jay was very knowledgeable about the medical aspects. I knew that they would both be good resources during my IVF process and had already begun to talk with them.

I made the long distance call to Florida, where Star had moved from Brooklyn.

"Hey, Star."

"Any news yet?"

"No. I'm still waiting."

"I remember when Jay and I waited each time until it finally worked. It was agony. The whole process was really stressful. Are you and Gabriel still getting along?"

"Yes. We're both really wanting it to work."

"What about the girls?"

"They are both praying it doesn't work."

"Do you want to speak with Jay too?"

"Okay."

"I wish you well on the pregnancy test. Maybe you'll be one of the really, really lucky ones."

It was time to have my blood drawn for the official pregnancy test. I was sure the results would be negative, but my daughter Lisette tried to be encouraging. She said, "You never know, Mom. Don't give up hope. Maybe you are pregnant."

I was at the Thai restaurant getting takeout dinner when my cell phone rang. It was my husband Gabriel with the results.

"The test shows you're pregnant."

"I'm pregnant!" I screamed in the middle of the restaurant as if I'd just won a game show. Then, for more privacy, I went to the vestibule at the front of the restaurant. This was a small space wedged between the two sets of glass entry doors. Once there, I heard Gabriel qualify the results. "Well, you're sort of pregnant. The lab and the hospital count pregnant as an hCG number of five or above.

You're pregnant but you're only a 19. You should have a value of about 50. In two days you'll have another test to make sure you are still pregnant. The number should at least double."

Well, I didn't know you could be a "little bit pregnant." As far as I was concerned the hospital and the lab criteria both considered me pregnant so I was pregnant. Yeahhh!

On the way home I passed in front of the Babies "R" Us store. I made a sudden swerve into the parking lot and got a spot right by the door. First I looked at all of the adorable outfits. There were cute tiny dresses with bows and little boy jumpsuits with matching hats. There also were beautiful blankets to take the baby home from the hospital. They even had diaper bags that looked like designer pocketbooks.

Then I looked at the bassinet section. The bassinets were very high-tech and performed multiple functions: they could play music, rock like a cradle, and become a changing table.

The best was the crib set. I fell in love with an "antique" one that looked like Victorian wrought iron, with a star and moon and a canopy on top. I started to call over the salesman to purchase it but managed to restrain myself.

Two days later I had my second blood test. While I was waiting for the results, Lauren called. She was pregnant with multiple children. Definitely more than two, but she didn't know how many yet—maybe enough for her to make it onto *Oprah*. She told me that the "hatching" really worked because a bunch of embryos latched on. Her husband was already worried about his multiple mouths to feed.

I was called again with my blood test result. The level had gone up to 31! It wasn't in the safe 50 zone, but it had almost doubled. The nurse said that the baby could make it, but the odds were slim. I had an image of the baby extending a little hand and trying to hold on tight to the wall of my womb. Every night I looked at my five fertilized eggs picture and wondered which was the baby struggling to make it. Finally I picked one egg and called him James. James became my child. He was fighting for his life. I was moving carefully, trying not to dislodge him. He would grow stronger with time. He would make it to his birth. Then Gabriel and I would take him home from the hospital, wrapped in his tiny blanket.

Brittany called me. Her pregnancy test was negative. Her sister

Dakota had already left for Australia. Brittany would fly back to London. They would try again in the summer. I lost Lauren's phone number and never found out if she eventually delivered her multiples.

By now I was bleeding. The doctor told me that some people bleed during pregnancy. The bleeding could even appear to be a period, but you could still be pregnant.

Two days later I went for the next pregnancy test. It was an anguished wait. This time when the nurse called she said the number had gone to 17. She said I should continue my progesterone shots because technically I was still pregnant. I knew that the numbers should be going up—not down. I asked to speak with a doctor. The doctor came on and said it was all over. Don't take any more progesterone shots. In fact the number 17 could be much lower and the baby might already have died, although I was still registering pregnant.

I felt the tears welling up and believed that they would never stop. I felt as if my baby was being ripped out from me. He had been there, trying so hard to make it. And now James was gone. The sense of emptiness was total.

I waited for Gabriel to return from work.

"Gabriel, the baby is gone."

"Oh no. I'm so sorry."

We hugged each other.

"What if we never have a baby?" said Gabriel.

"Don't worry. We'll try again. We'll have one."

Gabriel also had been positive that the IVF trial would work. He already had researched obstetricians and made me an appointment with one of the best in our area. He had also compiled a list of pediatricians.

Lisette told me I could always try again. If we came upon baby goods stores, she took my hand and pulled me quickly past them. She was relieved there was no baby but concerned about me.

Elizabeth asked me the result of each blood pregnancy test. She wanted to know the baby's progress and to provide reports to her friends. When there was no more baby, she wasn't surprised.

I did not want Elizabeth to tell everyone about my IVF trial. But I did not think it was right to dictate that it was a "family secret." Elizabeth probably needed to talk with her friends to help her cope with the whole situation. During my IVF trial, Elizabeth had also become a "mother." Her home economics class conducted mock marriages. Every girl was assigned a male classmate as her groom. They designed wedding invitations and chose their honeymoon spots. Then the lucky couples received an instantaneous family—two eggs with their contents blown out. The blushing bride cared for one egg, and her husband for the sibling. Both children had the husband's last name. Fortunately Elizabeth liked the partner in her arranged marriage.

Each day Elizabeth transported her egg baby, "Skyler Rose," to and from school in a shoebox. Skyler wore a miniature felt diaper and snuggled under a cotton ball blanket. Alas, Elizabeth had bad luck. The last day that Skyler was due back in class, Elizabeth tripped on the way to school, and Skyler became Humpty Dumpty.

Elizabeth had no second chances. I planned to keep trying.

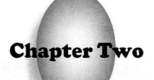

Chapter Two

No Spring Chicken

Doctor Shopping – February 2003

had a follow-up, failed-pregnancy appointment with my doctor. This was the first time that I had spoken with or met with
him since our initial meeting. He told me, "You had a chemical
pregnancy. It did not progress to the point where you could hear
a heartbeat." Matter-of-fact, he explained that the baby must have
been genetically defective. It all came down to the age of my eggs:
even if I managed to deliver a live baby, there was an increased risk
the baby would have something wrong with it. I would rather have
heard something about how sorry he was about my loss. To me it
was a true baby rather than a chemical occurrence.

This time I was prepared with my own research. I told him that I
had seen an article in the *New York Times* about a procedure in China
in which they kept the woman's nucleus from her egg but placed it in
a younger egg with its own nucleus removed. This technique could be
helpful for older women because the outer egg would still be young
and the genes would still be your own. However, the procedure was
now outlawed in China and already had been outlawed in the United
States because it was too close to the steps needed for cloning.

The doctor told me that this procedure was not perfected and
was not being done any more. However, in the future he thought
the answer would be in stem cells and the ability to utilize the genetic material from a woman's stem cell combined with the sperm
to create a viable embryo no matter what the age of the woman.

Unfortunately, it could take many years to perfect this procedure, which would not become available in time for me to benefit from it.

In the meantime, the answer for me was still a donor egg. The doctor told me again that they had an excellent donor egg program. I would need to go on a waiting list. The donor could be matched to look like me. In fact he had a colleague whose child looked just like his wife because of a well-matched donor egg. There would be a questionnaire for the donor to complete. At the conclusion of our meeting, he handed me donor egg pamphlets and told me to consider it seriously. My chances with a donor egg would be 50 to 60 percent, whereas chances with my own eggs were 9 percent or less. I should decide soon because with my own egg the cutoff age was forty-four. I would turn forty-five shortly, but the hospital would let me continue at forty-five since I had already started in the program. The cutoff for using someone else's egg in the donor program was forty-five. Although technically a woman could bear donor eggs at a later age there were other issues, such as staying alive through the growing years of your child.

I actually did start to consider the possibility of donor eggs. My first fantasy was to forget having the child matched to me. Why not choose a donor who looked like a model and was brilliant? If I was going to raise a child that was genetically not mine, why not pick an "ideal child"? However, I quickly thought better of this fantasy. If I was willing to accept my own genetic child, with whatever flaws, why should a donor one have to be so perfect? I should be ready to accept my child no matter what and not have double standards because in some ways it was "someone else's child."

Then there was the issue of the person donating. The questionnaire asked about her medical history and her family background. Yet what was to stop the woman from not telling the truth? Anyone who wanted to sell her eggs would hardly disclose that half her relatives were in jail and the other half hospitalized with schizophrenia.

Another question was the woman's motivation. I knew from firsthand experience that it was a major hardship to undergo hormone injections, sonograms, blood monitoring, anesthesia, an operation, and the possibility of life-threatening side effects such as hyperstimulation. Who would do that? A woman desperate for money, perhaps for a good cause such as caring for her ill father or her starving family … or perhaps to support a drug addiction. Maybe she would do it out of the goodness of her heart, to help others who were childless. Or because she wanted to populate the world with her own genetic children. I would never know the reason because I could not meet her, contact her, or even have her picture. Yet this stranger would have conceived the baby with my husband.

I thought about the testimonials from women who had been successful with donor eggs. They wrote about the joy of having a baby at last. However, they also wrote about a sense of loss (sometimes years later) that the child was not biologically their own.

I did not want to feel a sense of loss each time I looked at my "donor egg" child. I realized I would have to be at the point of total acceptance of this child, and I was not there yet. My hormone levels were good, my egg production was bountiful, I had achieved at least a "chemical" pregnancy. Why give up now? Gabriel agreed to try one more time with my eggs because we had come close with our chemical pregnancy. I was cocky. Last time I was pregnant for a short while. My body just needed a jumpstart. After all, I hadn't carried a baby for ten years. This time I would maintain my pregnancy for all nine months.

Six months later we tried again and failed. I was devastated. As we rebounded from this latest failure, however, our thoughts about how to go forward diverged.

My husband now was ready to go to the egg donor option. My chances would increase sixfold, he pointed out. Also why spend so much money on what was probably a lost cause? The odds were poor. However, I still wanted to go forward again with my own eggs.

I called Star for support. "Star, I can't believe it didn't work either time. Gabriel wants an egg donor but I want to try again with my eggs."

"Why don't you try a different doctor? You could use ours. He was great. He knew when my eggs were ready and got us Jewel. Plus he's a really nice guy."

I decided to look into it. If this doctor worked for Star, maybe he would work for me. I called another friend of mine, whom I had met in graduate school when she was studying nursing. She was married to an obstetrician.

"Carol, have you ever heard of this doctor that my friend recommended for me?"

"Have I heard of him? My husband got him his job! We got him to leave your previous doctor and to come to work with my husband. If we hadn't moved, my husband would still be there too!"

"Is he good? Is it worth switching hospitals and trying him out?"

"Definitely switch. He's also a great guy. Tell all of them hi and that you were in my wedding party."

"I will. Thanks, Carol."

I expected the doctor's office to roll out the red carpet when I told them about my wedding connection. Instead, the nurses said that I still needed the right FSH level. Luckily my FSH was even lower this time. It went from 6 to 5. I still had decent scores and was a viable candidate!

This new doctor was much more personable than the first one. He firmly shook my hand and my husband's hand. He made eye contact. When we told him that it was my second marriage and my husband's first, he confided that he too had been divorced and remarried.

We told him that we'd had one chemical pregnancy and one total failure. He made me feel good when he pointed out that my chart indicated no roadblocks. I responded well to medication, made a lot of eggs, and had good hormone levels. He said that many forty-five-year-old women didn't respond to medication or were perimenopausal. I felt pride in the youthfulness of my body. Then, however, he mentioned that, because of my age, my odds were still in the single digits. Still, because I had no other problems, it was possible that I could be one of the "forty-somethings" who fell into the small percentage of successful pregnancies. I immediately focused on my possibility for success.

I also was happy that the doctor took a different approach in my case, since I was such a good responder. We would skip the Lupron period. Once I got my natural period, I would come in the next day and immediately start hormones. Then, when my follicles were the appropriate size, the eggs would be removed. If possible the transfer of the embryos would wait until day five, the blastocyst stage. Perhaps this time I would actually make it to a day-five transfer! I was optimistic.

The doctor did try to restrain my optimism. He cautioned me that the process was still likely to fail, that I shouldn't try more than once or twice with my own eggs. After that, he felt, the odds of success probably decreased. Like my previous doctor, he said that my chances if I used a donor egg would jump to 50 to 60 percent. He didn't have to be much of a gambler to prophesy that I would fail, since my odds were in the single digits. Still, I planned to be in the 9 percent or less of women who were successful. Why shouldn't I be? After all, I had no other fertility issue except age.

I still felt that I would be lucky. It was my basic life philosophy that even if the next woman had an infertility twister raging inside her womb, mine was protected. It was like thinking that if a tree lands on a car during a storm, it will be the other driver and not you. I felt protected from inclement life events by a "lucky caul." I believed that in the end even undesirable events would turn into something positive.

My husband wasn't so optimistic. He strongly favored going with the 50 or 60 percent choice. However, because I really wanted my own egg and because this doctor was going to try something a little bit different, my husband went along.

The institution my new doctor was affiliated with required that I have a hysterosalpingogram to make sure that everything was in order for making babies. This test required lying on a table, putting my legs in the stirrups, and having pink dye shot throughout my reproductive system for about a half hour. This pretty-in-pink procedure can cause cramping, but I only felt mild tightening. The most serious complication is infection, which can necessitate removal of the fallopian tubes and therefore cause infertility. In my case, the doctor who carried out my test said that to him everything looked good, a result that was later confirmed by my new IVF doctor.

The day after my natural period started, I took public transportation to my new IVF hospital. I signed in on the same white sheet as everyone else. In fact when I arrived, I was the only person there! I went right to the back room to have my blood drawn. There was only one row of cubicles, and three different nurses asked if they could help me! This was fine service, without the wait. However, I was a little worried that no one else was there. What if there was something the matter with the place? Then I reminded myself that this was a known institution.

The nurse explained that I would be called that afternoon. If my blood levels were good, I would start my hormones that night.

Otherwise I would be delayed. "For a day or two?" I asked. "No," she replied. "If your levels aren't good, you'll have to wait for your next period to begin the trial."

The nurse informed me that my medication would be Gonal F, which I had used before, and Repronex, which was new to me. Both medications could be given subcutaneously in the abdomen (yeah!). Then I would return in five days for my next blood levels and sonogram. Five days! This was great. If I didn't have to come back for five days and my eggs were ready for retrieval on day fourteen, as they were for my last trial, then I was almost halfway done! I was thrilled to bypass as many shots, sonograms, Lupron periods, and waiting time as possible. Compared to the long lines of my other hospital, this was like celebrity service baby making. Later I learned my blood levels were satisfactory.

Five days after my hormones started, I was back for my second blood test and my first sonogram. After the blood test, I was led into the inner waiting room. This "room" consisted of two rows of chairs facing each other in an area wedged between the financial and blood-drawing sectors. The nurse apologized that I might have to wait up to ten minutes.

I began a conversation with a woman named Cindy. Like me, she had previously utilized the other doctor and hospital. In her case, however, the doctor never told her to use donor eggs. She was a good responder like me but three years younger. I guessed that early forties versus mid-forties made the difference. She preferred the nurses from the other institution and had undergone eight prior trials. Now, of her own choice, she was using a donor egg. Since the previous place wouldn't let her bring in her own donor, she had come here instead.

"My donor didn't even have an agent!" exclaimed Cindy. Cindy had flown her in from South Carolina. She explained that they both had blonde hair, but otherwise they didn't look alike; she told me the donor was also bright and looking for a job.

Of course I thought immediately: Why would she donate her eggs unless she needed the money? Her donor was in the waiting room at this very moment, Cindy said.

I was called for my sonogram and had to leave. The doctor said that my follicles were growing nicely and that my eggs would probably be ready for retrieval in five or six days. I was shocked. The whole cycle from my period to egg retrieval was going to take only ten or eleven days.

As I was leaving, I saw Cindy right before me. Curious, I followed her back into the waiting room and looked to see the donor she'd picked up. I couldn't believe it! She was like my fantasy model of a donor. The woman was about six feet tall, with fine, angular features and platinum blonde hair. She looked as if she'd come right off the pages of *Vogue* magazine! Cindy was right. Other than the blonde hair, they looked nothing alike.

I enjoyed talking with Cindy. It was helpful for me in going through this process, and it was too isolating to focus on nothing but Henry VIII and his wives. However, I felt conflicted because these people did not realize that snippets of their conversation might be repeated in a book I hoped to write about my IVF experiences (albeit under different identities). For the first time in almost thirty years I recalled a caricature drawn of me at my friend's Sweet Sixteen party. The artist who'd been hired to entertain us asked what I wanted to be when I grew up. An author, I replied. The caricaturist proceeded to draw an extremely unflattering rendition of me with the caption, "Watch what you say—you might be in one of my books one day!" Now, the prophecy was coming true, even if neither of us imagined I'd be quoting conversations about people's eggs!

Another time at the hospital, a woman was smiling at me.

I asked, "Are you at the tail end of your trial?"

She whispered very softly, "I'm pregnant."

The word "pregnant" was a red button, a trigger word for us desperately infertile women. Children were also a potential trauma. The last time I had waited for my sonogram in the inner sanctum, a woman arrived with an infant dressed in a frilly pink outfit and sat among us. The other women glared malevolently at both the woman and baby. Indeed, at the time our eggs were ready to be harvested and transferred, we received a notice informing us that out of consideration to the other patients, no children should accompany us at the time of either procedure.

Now, when Tammy told me she was pregnant, I replied with real enthusiasm. "That's great!"

It had taken her five trials to have her first child, she informed me. Now, on her second attempt, it had worked again, and it worked on the fourth trial. "The doctor came close, looked me right in the eye, and said, 'Use a donor egg,'" she said. Nonetheless, she had persisted with her own egg, and here she was pregnant at age forty-four! I was very encouraged. This was the best news I'd heard yet.

When I left the sonogram room, Tammy was waiting outside the door for me.

She said, "I have to make a confession. I am using a donor egg this time. I didn't want the other people to hear me in the waiting area." She then told me that she was keeping that fact a secret for three years. She had told her parents, friends, and her first child (from her own IVF egg) that the baby was totally hers. However, when her newborn turned three, she would first break the news to the donor egg child. Once the toddler heard the true story, Tammy would tell everyone else.

Oh, well, I thought: She's not the miracle example I'd hoped. It was still up to me to beat the odds and become the paragon of a forty-five-year-old miraculous conception.

At my next appointment I saw a pretty woman with almond-shaped blue eyes staring at me. Finally she came over.

"I love your pocketbook. That King Charles Spaniel on the bag is adorable. Do you have one?"

"I have a Shetland Sheepdog, but I bought the bag before I had a dog. I just liked the purse."

"Come on over and meet my husband. See, we were just looking at all the photos of our baby King Charles Spaniel."

I followed her to the corner of the waiting room.

"We are doing a co-culture now. This is our fifth IVF attempt. No luck yet," explained the wife.

The husband chimed in, "We'll keep going until it works. It's a numbers game. If you keep at it, eventually you'll get pregnant. It took Courtney Cox eight times, and Geena Davis got pregnant when she was forty-eight."

I guessed that their King Charles Spaniel desperately needed a human brother or sister.

At first this encounter made me think I should tell my husband we should keep trying with my own egg—at least eight times. Then it occurred to me we might all have to join a group called "IVF Anonymous." A bunch of us might even become homeless and broke because we refused to give up, certain that the next time we'd hit the jackpot of a beautiful baby. In my mind I imagined the waiting room contingent, dressed in tatters and looking like the beggars in Penn Station. I wished the couple good luck as my name was called.

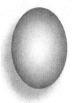

Hitting a Record Number: 1098

Five was still the magic number. Five days after my day-five sonogram, I was already at my egg retrieval. This pre-operation waiting room was an open area at the mezzanine level above the main waiting room. There were chairs along the walls and a table with a flyer about egg donation. At this hospital egg retrieval was organized by couples rather than by groups of three women.

Once again the husbands were called out one by one for their sperm donation. The husband after mine came back exclaiming, "Corny, corny, corny!" His wife asked him what was the matter. "The porn flicks are from the eighties!" he complained.

This hospital also had an operating table surrounded by bright lights that shined in my eyes. It was as if I were back on stage in my high school play. When I woke up, I immediately asked, "How many eggs?"

"Fourteen," replied the doctor. It was as if my entire self-worth was based on the number of eggs emerging from my follicle chicken coop.

Unfortunately, this was no day five for my egg transfer; the eggs would be returning on day three. When I arrived with my husband, we were the only people there. Once again it was like a ghost town. The doctor, a debonair Dr. Kildare, met with us first. The doctors rotated days, and so far I hadn't seen the same doctor twice. I was hoping to hear that a lot of eggs were being put back, but instead he told me that only one egg was really viable. It had divided six times and was not fragmented. Three other eggs had divided four times. The one "six-timer," he told me, was worth more than the other three put together. Still, he would be transferring all four.

On the way to the operating room, I warned the doctor that I was in the statistical group of one fifth of all women whose uterus was retroverted (faced backward, rather than forward). I wanted to make sure he didn't deposit my eggs in the wrong location. The doctor said not to worry. However, when he tried to put the eggs back, he couldn't reach the proper place. His next strategy, he said, was to "straighten" my uterus by pulling on the cervix. He utilized a clamp to pull, and I looked at the ceiling and tried to think of something pleasant during this painful process. But I wasn't straightening out. Finally the doctor employed a bent catheter to counteract the slant of my uterus, and that finally worked.

The doctor wasn't sure if all four eggs had left the catheter but informed me that even if one of the "bad" eggs had been left behind, he wouldn't go back to place it and risk dislodging the one "good" egg. As things turned out, I was lucky and all four eggs were in place.

I was given the score card that provided a history of my fourteen eggs. At this hospital, I needed to fill out a form to request that an e-mail be sent to me with a photo of my eggs. I had already seen a picture of them on the big screen on the wall in the operating room. The doctor had pointed out the one good egg and described it as a flower. He showed me the unsightly bumps on the three fragmented eggs. "Scientifically speaking," he said, "these are the icky eggs."

With only one good egg, I was not hopeful that this pregnancy was going to succeed. However, that night I woke up nauseated. Could I already have morning sickness? Finally I fell back to sleep. In the morning I was still nauseated. Now I was optimistic—maybe my history of severe morning sickness made me feel nauseated immediately! I savored the nausea. I did not try to throw up. I did not even buy a box of crackers to alleviate it. I decided to call the nurse with the joyful news. Instantly she deflated my hopes: It was the progesterone shots that were making me nauseated, not an implanted embryo.

A week before the pregnancy test, the new institution wanted my progesterone level. Even though they didn't request it, I had the local lab also draw my estradiol level, remembering from Lauren that a high estradiol could mean a pregnancy.

Well, my progesterone came back higher than ever before—106. My estradiol, though, was incredible. It was 1,098! The only person I had known with levels like that was Lauren. First she had been at 500, and then over 1,000. Of course she was carrying multiples. I hoped I wasn't having twins or triplets, but at least I should be pregnant. Immediately I called the doctor on call. He told me that since their institution didn't draw blood for estradiol at that stage, he couldn't tell me the meaning of the result.

Next I called a nurse from my previous IVF hospital. I asked her what a progesterone level of 106 and an estradiol of 1,098 might mean. I expected her to congratulate me on my baby. However, she couldn't even say definitively that I was pregnant, although she did say that a high estradiol level was a good sign. I asked if an estradiol could be over 1,000 without being pregnant. She wasn't sure. She did say that estrogen rose with the hCG level, which I knew was the pregnancy measure. Maybe my hCG was high since my estradiol was over 1,000. My next plan of action was to start the home pregnancy tests, even if it was too early. Perhaps I had such a phenomenally high level that I'd already register as pregnant.

Every day I used the home pregnancy test. Immediately I saw one pink line. Then I waited patiently for the second pink line that never appeared.

When the store ran out of the two pink lines test (I was probably their best customer), I bought a new test. On this one you waited for a blue cross: The vertical blue line materialized immediately, but you were pregnant only when the horizontal one showed up. When I first tried this test, I definitely saw a faint blue horizontal line. However, by the time I woke my husband excitedly the line was no longer there. It had probably been the angle of the morning light—or my desperation.

The next morning, before my lab test, I was ready with two home pregnancy tests. I demonstrated great dexterity. I created my own two-ring circus and simultaneously tried the blue and pink tests. In the first ring was a solitary blue line, and in the second a solitary pink one.

Not taking no for an answer, I decided to speak with the nurse on call. I told her that I had just performed two pregnancy tests and that

they were both negative. I said that I understood that it might be too
early to tell, but was it a bad sign?

This nurse was honest. She told me that urine tests were pretty ac-
curate. By now I should have a positive. A negative either meant that
I was not pregnant or that I had a low value of hCG, which must be
carefully monitored. I knew all about the low value hCG result already
from my prior "chemical" pregnancy. I hopped into the car to drive to
the local lab, convinced now about the negative result.

Nothing! Nothing! There was nothing at all. All promising numbers had flat-lined. The record 1,098 estradiol was now less than 20,
and the 106 had plummeted to 29. The most important number, the
hCG level, was less than 2. There was no baby, and if there ever had
been one it hadn't lasted long enough this time to leave even a chemical mark.

I was plunged back into my black hole.

Chapter Three

Humpty Dumpty Clung to the Wall

Game Plan—January 2004

I had to crawl out of the hole and begin again. The "Energizer" egg maker, always powered to go! First there was the phone consultation to discuss the failed trial. The doctor told me that I still could try one more time. The worse quality of these last eggs was not necessarily because of my age. My 1,098 estradiol level could have meant that I was pregnant and lost the baby. It also might have meant absolutely nothing.

I later discussed the phone consultation with Gabriel.

"Gabriel, we can try again. The doctor says my eggs could be better next time."

"Victoria, what's the point? We've already tried three times. It's time for an egg donor."

"I want to try again with my eggs. The doctor already said we could try a couple of times. We're not done yet. If it doesn't work next time, then I'll agree to a donor. Gabriel, if it doesn't work with my egg, or a donor, then would you want to adopt?"

"No."

"Why?"

"I just wouldn't."

"That's because you don't want someone else's sperm."

I knew that he wouldn't elaborate because he wouldn't admit his double standard—he didn't mind if it wasn't my egg so long as it was his sperm. He ruled out the adoption option because he wanted a genetic child.

Admittedly, I too wanted my own genetic egg. True, I had now agreed to try an egg donor next time, but I was praying hard I wouldn't really have to face that possibility. The donor egg route was where Gabriel and I parted ways. It was his best hope and my very last resort.

Once again I had to break the no-baby news to everyone. This time Elizabeth, just thirteen, had also been rooting for a baby and was disappointed that the trial didn't work. She wanted it to succeed so that we could move. If I had a baby, there wouldn't be enough bedrooms in our house, and she wanted to be first to pick her new bedroom.

"Elizabeth, I have bad news."

"You're not pregnant."

"No, it didn't work."

"Now I'll never get my new room."

Next I approached Lisette, almost eleven, with the news. "Lisette, I'm not pregnant."

"Why do you want a baby anyway? We don't need one. You have me."

My parents were as unenthusiastic about a baby as Lisette. "I'm sorry that it didn't work. Victoria, you should give up now. I hope you're finished. You've tried your hardest and now it's time to walk away," advised my mom.

"I'm not done yet."

"Victoria, these treatments will kill you. If you ever get a tumor the hormones will make it spread like wildfire. Besides you could incur permanent damage from a pregnancy at your age."

"It could be very dangerous to your health," added my father.

I was willing to face the breakdown of my body for the reward of giving birth to Gabriel's child with my own egg.

I also shared the news with Star.

"Victoria! Are you pregnant?"

"No. It didn't work."

"I'm truly sorry. I really thought my doctor could help you."

"Well, he was really nice. It just didn't work."

"How are you and Gabriel taking it?"

"We're both really upset."

"How is your marriage going?"

"We don't agree anymore. I want to still use my eggs and he wants a donor."

"Jay and I were fighting a lot during the whole process. We went to a marriage counselor."

"I haven't refused to use a donor, so it isn't all-out war yet."

To help me handle the loss from my last failed attempt and the stress of what would happen next, I turned to eBay, and for two weeks I became an eBay addict. Rather than checking pregnancy tests, I followed my auction bids.

When I lived upstate, where antiquing was cheap, I had purchased serving pieces from a Victorian silver-plated tea set, each piece of which featured a regal lion holding a shield. Now my eBay treasure trove was other pieces with lions. First I discovered a maple syrup pitcher with a lion. I entered the fray with my highest bid amount and won my prize. Next I spent a week fighting for a napkin ring with my lion. I became victorious at every battle by raising my bid, and the napkin ring was conquered. Boxes of eBay booty began arriving at my doorstep.

My final prize was an ornate butter dish with scrollwork, etched flowers, and the requisite king of beasts. This item had the "buy it now" option. But why buy it now when the bidding started at $9.99? I watched the item until the end. At one minute before the auction terminated, I entered my final highest amount (still below the "buy it now" option) and went to bed. When I woke up, I went to check my e-mail. Instead of the bill, I received a "you were outbid" notice. According to my brother, Mark, an eBay expert, I had been "sniped"— someone had come online out of the blue, a few seconds before the auction ended, and outbid me.

I decided to walk away from eBay. I did not want my entire house to be covered with lion teapots. I would have to deal with my feelings of loss without going on a perpetual shopping spree.

Anyway I was back in the fray one more time with my own eggs. The doctor on duty at my appointment was a slender woman whose body did not look as if it had ever been pregnant. She was having a busy day and complained, "Boy, everyone must be starting their period. Something must be going on—everyone is in sync today!" I said it was nothing compared to the crowd at my prior institution! She told me that I should write a book about the two places that provided an insider's perspective on the city's two premier IVF sites. She also told me that my sonogram indicated that "the runway was clear."

The *New York Times* that day reported an unexpected discovery: female mice could actually make new eggs from their ovarian stem cells. Here was the sign that eventually, with new research, science might be able to encourage the production of new eggs from the stem cells of the ovaries of older women. Right now, however, we were still at the beginning stage of learning about mice. This research was going to be too late to help me, of course.

Yet I couldn't help feeling that sliver of hope. If the mice could make new eggs, maybe I could too! Perhaps not all of my eggs were the ones that I was born with—the ones that had been on the shelf too long and turned to vinegar. After all, I was only getting one type of hormone, Follistim, no Pergonal or Repronex. Wasn't that a good sign I had strong baby making machinery? Last time I had been on Gonol F instead of Follistim. Further evidence of my fertility talents? No, the nurse informed me: Gonol F and Follistim were like "Coke and Pepsi"; they were interchangeable. Follistim went into the abdomen, not the rump (yeah!). However, I still needed two shots a day because the doctor wanted me to receive one dose of Follistim in the morning and one in the evening. Now I was awakened early each morning by my husband standing over my stomach with a big needle.

While my hospital trials continued, so did outside family life. Both of my children act as a hobby, and they both had an agent who periodically sent them on auditions. The mother of another child actress had recommended that I buy *Back Stage* magazine, which listed casting calls and other auditions my children could go to independent of the agent, even if the agent still received her 10 percent commission.

My younger child, Lisette, had just been in a movie shown at the Sundance Film Festival, and she was in a union commercial that paid her residuals. My older daughter, Elizabeth, had callbacks to be a lead in two films. One film, *The Woodsman*, required a lot of dramatic ability because she would have to play an abused child. However, Elizabeth had yet to be booked for any films.

I decided to buy the magazine. There were no appropriate casting calls for children their age. However, there were competing ads, one of which stated, "We Are Looking for Extraordinary Women to Do Something Extraordinary." Also prominently displayed was the compensation fee: $7,500. The headline for another ad: "Your Chance to Make a Difference." In bold numbers underneath was the figure "$7,000."

These were ads to become an egg donor. Two hospitals were vying to attract actress donors. The money was much better than waitressing. An actress could donate for years while waiting to land a breakout role. The chances of becoming a star were probably no better than the single-digit odds of a forty-something-year-old woman becoming a mother with her own egg. *Back Stage* magazine provided a financial link between the two populations.

It was then that I remembered an article in the *New York Times* about *Back Stage* that said that Southern Baptists, to attract new converts among disillusioned actors, had been advertising in the magazine. Both those in need of eggs and those pursuing an increased religious congregation had turned to the actors of America.

As one way to escape the tension over the IVF trial, Gabriel and I went to see the Broadway show *Gypsy*. It was intermission, and I was on a huge bathroom line. I began to feel nauseated. Then I felt lightheaded. I knew I was close to fainting.

I told the woman ahead of me, "My name is Victoria Hopewell. I think I'm going to faint. Please have them call for my husband, Gabriel, if I faint."

The woman said, "No speak English, no speak English!"

The next thing I knew I was on the floor surrounded by people.

I really felt sick and pleaded, "I need a garbage bag because I think I'm going to throw up."

Someone brought the entire garbage pail, filled with garbage, from the ladies' room. I started to vomit into the garbage. A little later everyone left: either my throwing up drove them away or it was the start of the second act. My husband arrived shortly after. Perhaps someone else on the line who spoke English had overheard me.

The medics arrived, and I stayed in the bathroom lounge for the second act of the play. The next day I had an echocardiogram and an electrocardiogram. I also wore a Holter to monitor my heart. Everything was "normal." The doctor concluded that I had had a case of food poisoning and was prone to "vasovagal response" (fainting).

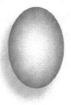

Waxing My Legs

W hen I woke from egg retrieval a week or so later, I was totally disoriented. I did not realize that I was in the hospital. In the background I could hear Bernadette Peters singing "Everything's Coming Up Roses," and for a moment I thought that I was at a Broadway play and that I had just fainted. It took a moment for me to realize that I wasn't back in the ladies' room at *Gypsy*, but in the recovery room ready for the next scene of my own drama. As I collected myself, the imperative question came immediately. "How many eggs this time?" The answer was sixteen.

Three days later, it was time to put the eggs back. An hour and a half before train time, I looked down upon my legs in horror. It was the winter, a time I took the lax approach of walking around with hairy legs because no one saw them anyway. Today, however, was the egg transfer day. I had visions of a scene out of *Seinfeld* when I was lying unconscious on the operating table on Friday and the doctors were discussing my unsightly ape legs. Well, I thought: I won't just shave, I'll show up at my transfer with squeaky clean waxed legs.

I jumped in the car and went to a beauty salon. It was closed. So I went to the one across the street. It was open, but the person who waxes didn't come in on Mondays. Then I went downtown to a nail salon that had just opened. Yes, they did waxing. I lay down on the table and waited to get waxed. I was in the back room with the curtains drawn around me—good practice for the hospital recovery bed.

I was assigned the "waxer in training." First she put a spot of wax on my leg. She took an adhesive white cloth and put it on the wax. She lifted it up and looked at the cloth. There was not much hair on the cloth. Then she repeatedly put the cloth on the same spot over and over. The supervisor came to check and showed her how to press the cloth down firmly over the wax.

Then the new waxer grabbed the tweezers. She dug them into my leg and tried to reach for the "short" hairs. Painstakingly she tweezed all hairs from a small area of my leg. Then the supervisor returned to inspect. She pointed out a few missed hairs from that region. This process was repeated over and over for each zone of my leg.

My anxiety started to build. What if I missed the train because I was having my legs waxed? Suddenly it seemed ridiculous even to worry about the doctors seeing hairy legs—they would be focusing instead on getting the eggs back. Worrying about my hairy legs was as absurd as worrying about what underwear you were wearing before you leaped off a bridge. And being gouged with the tweezers wasn't a relaxing activity to prepare me for egg transfer.

Finally I jumped off the table. "I don't care if you missed some hairs. I have to leave for a doctor's appointment in the city," I told them and I dashed to the station with five minutes to spare.

Luckily I made it to the transfer on time. I was in the changing room in front of a row of lockers. I dumped my belongings in one of the lockers, locked it, and placed a yellow elastic band with a key on my wrist. As I was undressing, a sobbing woman burst into the room. She was still wearing her cloth cap and her dark curls poked out from under, making her look like Betsy Ross or a tour guide from Colonial Williamsburg.

"I'm sorry, I didn't know you were in here. I was going to change. I just got my eggs back today on the fifth day, and I'm so emotional. To-morrow I'll hear if any of the eggs get frozen," explained the woman.

"If they went to the fifth day and they might freeze some, they have to be wonderful eggs."

Her name was Madison, the woman told me, and she smiled for the first time. "You have made me so happy. I'm really glad to get this information. I didn't know any of it."

In the waiting room later, Madison's husband came over and

thanked me for cheering up his wife. He was a handsome man with finely formed features.

"You seem so strong," Madison said.

"It's because I've done it before," I said. I felt like Lauren. After four trials, I'd become a kind of maven of IVF.

The doctor, with thin lips, called me into the little consulting room near the operating room. "Hi! I'm Victoria. I assume that there's something to put back if I'm here. I just hope there's something decent. Last time out of fourteen eggs, only one was really any good," I nervously explained. The doctor reassured me that there were five eggs ready for transfer. One was a grade one and another was a grade two that had divided nine times. I was ecstatic. I'd never had the highest, grade one egg, and I'd never had an egg with nine cell divisions.

I told the doctor, "I'm so glad that my eggs were good this time. I was worried that they'd gotten worse with age because of my poor eggs last time."

The doctor chillingly replied, "Someone should explain to you the difference between eggs that appear to be good externally and those that have internally decayed from age."

For a moment my hopes were dashed. I remembered what my original doctor had told me about a patient in her forties who always made beautiful, grade one eggs that fertilized and divided but never led to pregnancies. Externally her eggs were flawless, but internally defective. Well, I would show these doctors! My eggs would be excellent quality and genetically intact. I was one woman whose eggs you could judge by their covers!

Although I still wasn't using the Lauren approach of taking the week off after the transfer, I had taken some steps to decrease my load of stress. When I married Gabriel, my daughters and I relocated, since our Long Island town would have been a difficult, "over the bridge" commute for Gabriel. Instead, now I was going over the bridge from Westchester. Twice a week I still traveled to my private practice. I had consolidated the evening hours into two full days. In the meantime I was building a practice near my new home. I also obtained local, part-time employment to do psychological testing. Every IVF trial had coincided with this one-day-a-week testing job. The woman who had hired me had taken six months to make her decision. First she had wanted every letter of recommendation that I could find; then she had called everyone on the long list of phone numbers I provided, including a friend from graduate school. My friend Joanna informed me that talking to this woman had been the Inquisition, and warned me against working for her—she would claim your soul, she predicted.

When I started work, naturally, right when I was beginning my first IVF trial, my new boss told me we were already behind with six months of backlogged work. Of course, I thought to myself, because you waited six months to hire me.

The woman had the boundaries of an amoeba. She called at eleven at night, on weekends, and on holidays. She called on my cell phone, home phone, and work phone. She told me to come in on Sunday, pick something up from the typist at ten p.m., work on Memorial Day, and meet with people at night. During every IVF trial, I heard her voice on my machine with a new demand. As soon as I recognized it, I cringed.

Finally, before my final IVF trial, I decided to quit. I told the woman that my own practice hours were increasing and that I no longer had time to work for her. "Well, it really wasn't working for me either," she replied. "I need to be in total control. I must know what people are doing at all times and know that my employees are always available. You weren't available enough."

At last I was no longer working for this woman, and life was relatively calm. The day the nurse told me I was a prime candidate for implantation, I was taking it easy. That night I came home and played my messages. There was that woman's voice again. She was demanding that I immediately pick up the final test report the typist had just completed. "You'd better be an adult and get that report," she insisted. Immediately I picked up the phone. It was ten p.m., but I broke my own rule of not calling anyone at that hour.

My voice was shaking. "I want you to know that I just had two surgical procedures. I also would like to point out that I wrote that report weeks ago, and you just gave it to the typist now. I went beyond the call of duty, and I'm very insulted by what you said on the phone."

The woman apologized, explaining that she had been "overwhelmed and acted inappropriately." It was too late. My stomach was churning. Once again the eggs would have a uterine rollercoaster ride.

Informing my private patients when I'd be out also brought a level of stress. IVF and work were not a good combination. The bloodlettings, sonograms, retrievals, and transfers were not on a set schedule. To my patients, I said only that I was having "medical procedures" that had to be scheduled at the last moment. I reassured them all that it was "nothing serious." Of course to me it was dead serious and my major focus.

I also was becoming more and more isolated. It was difficult to see any friends and hard to carry on a luncheon conversation. I became obsessed about whether this time I would have Grade A eggs. My mood was anxious and depressed, and I wasn't as good a listener for my girlfriends.

Once I had an "early morning" awakening. The one remaining pregnancy test from my prior IVF trials was next to my bed in the night table drawer. This time I wanted to wait until the actual blood test. However, it was five days before my real test day, and the earliest date designated on the pregnancy test. My hands were twitching by my side as I lay in bed. Finally I could resist no longer. I grabbed the pregnancy test and dashed to the bathroom.

I watched the liquid turn pink as it rose to the level of the clear plastic window. The single pink line appeared, and I waited for the second crucial line to materialize.

During this IVF trial I was reading about the children of Henry VIII. Henry's oldest child, Mary, conceived with Catherine of Aragon, had two "pregnancies." Both times her periods ceased, her stomach extended, and she went into confinement waiting for a baby that never appeared. Mary wanted a baby so much that she had two psychosomatic pregnancies.

My level of belief was strong too. I savored every moment of nausea. I stared hard at that plastic white stick, willing that second pink line to appear. The harsh white light of the bulb in the bathroom revealed the sad truth: there was no line. Still, I decided to buy more pregnancy tests and repeat this test of faith every morning.

On the fifth day, however, I did not buy the final home pregnancy test. Instead I decided to sit and wait for the official pregnancy call.

The cell phone rang. No one was there. It was a voice message.

"Hi. I'm calling with your pregnancy results. You are not pregnant. I repeat, the results are negative. That means you are not pregnant. If you want to pursue this further you can call the doctor." This was the least personal message yet. If I had wanted to shoot the messenger, I would have had to jump up and down on my cell phone. This time there was no sinking feeling. I'd already cried during all the negative home pregnancy tests. I sensed it was over when I recognized the symptoms of my upcoming period. I spent days knowing that I would never have another blood child. Now I was numb.

Chapter Four

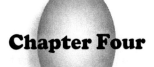

Donor Egg Hunt

Where's My Uterus?—March 2004

I would have to uphold my end of the bargain. I promised my husband a donor egg trial, and I would keep my promise. I still expected one of my own eggs to ride in on a white steed, dressed in a suit of armor, and rescue me from the fate of a surrogate egg. Unfortunately, I didn't hear any hoofbeats. Underneath I felt tremendous sadness.

When Gabriel finally returned from work, I heard more of his reaction to our latest negative pregnancy result. "Victoria, it just wasn't meant to be. We really gave it our all. They just don't have the technology for us yet to make it work."

Gabriel was not as sad as after the other three failed attempts. Now he had a much greater chance of siring a ninth-generation descendant, even a female one, in honor of his famous family holy ancestor. I did not want to be the one responsible for ending his bloodline. I wasn't terminating the genetic pool of a great inventor like Thomas Edison or a mathematical genius like Albert Einstein. But I would be stopping a Jewish spiritual connection. Many of my grandmother's first cousins perished in the Holocaust. Perhaps providing another link to Gabriel's revered Jewish ancestor was a way of honoring my own murdered Jewish relatives who had never had the chance to procreate. The time of donor egg had arrived. Gabriel knew that I would keep my promise and increase our odds of success.

My brother Mark called to say that he was sorry; he also shared his skepticism about the entire idea. "Victoria, I would never want a baby now. How could you think of starting again? Maybe Gabriel wants one, but I can't imagine that you would." Like my father, he saw me as sacrificing my life for the sake of a new baby.

Next I told the children that my IVF had not worked.

Lisette was angry. "You should stop. You don't want a baby anyway. You're just doing it for Dad. You never cared about having a baby before. Besides Dad won't have any time to be with the baby."

Lisette did have a point. Gabriel was hardly ever home. Our first year together, he had consistently returned home from work in time for dinner, and I had tried to hone my nonexistent cooking skills to prepare meat and chicken dishes with elaborate sauces. Gabriel was an internist at a hospital. He saw both inpatients and outpatients. There were life-threatening emergencies, but the fellows and residents handled the middle-of-the-night crises.

Our second year of marriage, everything changed. Gabriel had two physician co-workers. One of them dropped dead of a heart attack while on the job (probably from work stress) and the other one never came back from her pregnancy leave. No new replacements were hired, and Gabriel had to work overtime. On a good night he might return home at nine p.m. His employers were hunting for another doctor, but they weren't looking very hard. After all, Gabriel's performing the job of three for the price of one was a great deal for them!

When Gabriel wasn't working, he divided his time between us and his parents. Some weekends he went to New Jersey to sleep over at his parents' apartment. He would take them to Saturday doctor appointments, buy them a huge supply of groceries, and help them to pay bills.

Lisette wanted Gabriel to be around more. Elizabeth was locked in her room listening to music and was not concerned about spending additional time with any of her parents. I was happy that Gabriel still displayed the qualities of a mensch and helped his elderly parents. However, that did not stop me from being resentful that he could not be with us more.

Elizabeth also was angry about the pregnancy news. "Stop spending money," she said. "It won't work anyway. You could take all of the money and redo my room. We'll never move. There'll never be a baby.

So why not fix up the house?" The only good news was that Elizabeth had been booked for a part in a feature film.

I began to investigate egg donors. My second institution, the site of my last failed attempts, allowed egg donation up to age fifty. They targeted eggs from trade papers, with a focus on women who were looking for a job. They also ran a group for prospective egg recipients. I asked to attend the group. I was told that I couldn't attend the meeting until I was officially waitlisted as a potential egg recipient. The process started with a three-hour evaluation by a psychologist. I also checked to see if my first hospital ran a group. I was informed that there was no group, because their egg donor recipients wanted to be totally anonymous and did not want anyone to find out that the eggs weren't their own.

Both hospital programs evaluated the potential donor for disease. They did not want to give you a donor egg from someone with HIV, for example. The second program could try to match a hobby of the donor to your own interest but printed a disclaimer in their pamphlet that interests had been shown not to be genetic. I didn't care whether the donor liked stamp collecting or skateboarding, but I did prefer someone who was bright and had completed college.

I was embarrassed to inform the doctor that I cared about intelligence on my phone consultation. I was afraid of sounding elitist. The doctor then told me about the recent lawyer couple. They were both attorneys and had turned down a donor with a great record of having eggs carried by other women. However, this donor had a B average in school, and the lawyers wanted an A average egg. They waited three more months for "Grade A" eggs. That absurd story made me feel even more stupid for caring about intelligence.

I also told the doctor about the woman I had met in the waiting room with the attractive egg donor from South Carolina (I omitted the part about her looking like a model). I asked if there were ever issues about the donor wanting visiting rights to the child. He said that the donor and recipient work out the details, but that their program was anonymous and did not reveal the egg donor's identity. He had never heard of children who went searching for the woman who donated their eggs. In fact the doctor felt that few children would ever seek out such a donor anyway. He believed that children who were

adopted were motivated to find the parents who had in effect "rejected" them by giving them away. According to the doctor, there were no
such motivational factors with an egg donor. The child would realize
that this was simply the method that had enabled his or her parents to
have a baby, that the "egg mother" had just assisted with her donation.

My first hospital had eggs that came mainly from college students, so I decided to call them. I informed them that I was ready for
a donor egg. They told me that there was a waitlist for an egg. "Did I
want a Jewish egg?" I said it didn't matter. Well, then, I would have an
edge and move more quickly up the list. "Jewish eggs are in demand,"
explained the egg coordinator. I guessed that many Jewish people believed that the mother must be Jewish for the baby to be truly Jewish.

Initially my husband also had some concerns about Jewish eggs.
He researched the theological point involved. Fortunately, the book he
read quoted a rabbi who advised not to use Jewish eggs. A baby who
comes out of the loins of a Jewish woman becomes Jewish no matter
the religion of the donor, the rabbi proclaimed. In fact it could be a
sin to use Jewish eggs: After all, the donor might be a long-lost Jewish
relative, and then there would have been incest! With all this clarified,
we still could be high on the waitlist.

I returned to my original hospital. It was late afternoon, and the
place was deserted. There were no women patients and their husbands
jostling other couples to vie for the remaining seats, but I did see two
familiar faces. The young fellow in training, the one with the goatee,
was running down the hall. He remembered me and stopped to say
hello. The doctor who had aspirated my cyst with no anesthesia was
there momentarily, and he too greeted me with a smile.

My husband was caught in traffic. We were both supposed to meet
with the donor egg psychologist. The psychologist, who appeared very
professional in a business suit, kept peering into the waiting room and
looking at her watch. She said that if my husband didn't come soon,
the meeting would have to be canceled. Finally Gabriel arrived, just
before she lost all patience.

The psychologist took my husband and me into a private room.
She explained that there were a couple of issues to discuss about egg
donation. First, it was important for me to allow for a long period of
grieving the loss of my own biological child. We also needed to be

prepared for the repercussions of having a child at a later age. When we brought the child places, people would think we were the grandparents. At some point the laws might change and information about the egg donor might be available for our child to uncover. We must accept that possibility. Apparently the psychologist didn't agree with the doctor who had asserted that a donor child would not be motivated to find his or her biological egg mother. Finally, we must be ready for twins. In fact many donor recipients were delivering triplets. The hospital would perform "reductions" for triplets, but not twins. However, the new protocol was to place only two eggs to prevent triplets. The young eggs meant that, despite my older age, I was now as much at risk for multiples as a younger woman. Twins! I did not want twins. One was enough at age forty-six.

She said we could ask questions about the donors. I told her perhaps it was misguided, but I cared about intelligence. I explained that both of my biological children were very bright, and I would want this baby to be smart as well.

She replied, "Don't feel funny, in fact intelligence is the most requested characteristic."

I elaborated, "I understand your pool of donors comes from the local Ivy League college, the other local four-year college, which is a good school, and the associated medical school."

The psychologist was blunt. "Most of our donors have completed only high school. An Ivy League donor is the exception. If you want an Ivy League donor you should go to an agency. The agency pays fifty thousand to the donor, and we pay seven thousand. There are some agencies that will provide Ivy League eggs and photos of the donor. Your information will remain confidential. You might have to wait years for an Ivy League egg from our institution."

Well, I guess Ivy League donors were smart enough to locate places that paid more.

Next I showed her photos of me, my children, and my husband. I said I knew that donors could be matched to my facial features, or, if I requested it, to the features of my children. I pointed out the acting headshots that were closeups of my children's faces so that their appearance could be carefully taken into account as well. The psychologist stated nonchalantly that I could give the nurse one family photo on my way out. The donor would be matched to my eye and hair color.

The donor program was like a bad dating service with a limited pool of men. You could request different physical characteristics, but you could only be matched on eye and hair color.

I was crushed. I left the hospital in a daze. My husband brought me to the Metropolitan Museum of Art to cheer me up. It was my favorite museum, but I wandered around the exhibit of the glass-enclosed Egyptian mummies ready to burst into tears. Only the floor with the Impressionist paintings helped alleviate my mood a little.

I decided the party line would be "it's my egg." Family members would know the truth that it was really from a donor—maybe a few very select friends too, but that would be it.

Already I had become convinced that the whole town knew I was doing IVF trials. I had asked a friend who had a daughter Elizabeth's age not to tell anyone about my IVF. Yet when I was in the final week of waiting for my last pregnancy result, she approached me at our children's school. "You'll never guess!" she exclaimed. "Lulu from the PTA's cousin is using the same doctor as you for her IVF trial. She is only two days behind you. Lulu and I have been talking all about it." My heart sank. Normally I would have been happy to hear that someone else had my doctor. I even would have asked for her phone number. But not when I had told my friend not to tell! I had wanted to maintain a degree of privacy. I didn't want everyone asking me if I was pregnant yet, when in the end I might not even succeed. Now it was likely all the PTA mothers and everyone else Lulu and my friend had spoken to knew all my IVF trial details. This incident made me decide I would no longer be so open about my IVF attempts, especially egg donation. I did not want school board members to ring my doorbell with the welcome wagon for the first donor egg baby in the district.

One of my friends from graduate school actually asked me if I was using my own egg or a donor's. "I hope you don't mind my asking," she said. "You see, I have a friend who had twins last year with donor eggs, and I thought maybe you'd use a donor egg this time."

"So far I've only used my own eggs, but doctors have been talking to me about using a donor."

I was taken aback that she knew about donor eggs and that she asked me directly. Perhaps many people were egg savvy these days. As

I walked my baby to the park, would strangers ask if it was my egg or someone else's? I would have to prepare my answer to that question.

Shortly afterward my "mock trial" started. This time my injections, blood drawings, and sonograms would not produce a baby, but a piece of tissue. After I had gone through a natural period, ovulation, the start of Lupron shots, and then a Lupron period, the doctors would perform a biopsy on my uterine lining. If the uterine lining was thick, the donor egg would have an ideal place to rest once it was implanted. If it was suboptimal, I would need additional time (and shots) to achieve the desired consistency. My lining was the pie shell, and it must be thick enough to hold the mixture of egg and sperm before I could progress to the next step. Pie was on my mind because I had enjoyed Shoofly pie on an expedition to Lancaster, Pennsylvania, with the family over a recent Memorial Day weekend.

Lancaster was our "educational" trip. I remembered it because my parents had taken me there when I was ten. Families from New York, New Jersey, and Connecticut often drove the few hours to rural Pennsylvania to expose their children to another culture and time period. The Amish maintained practices and customs from the nineteenth century. They were forbidden to drive or ride in cars and to wear modern-day clothing.

Our pit stop at Dorney Amusement Park was successful. When we arrived in Lancaster, Elizabeth and Lisette were enthralled by the first three horse-and-buggies that rolled by and mesmerized by the Amish teens who rollerbladed down the lane. By the time Gabriel and I pointed to the tenth horse-and-carriage, however, their interest was gone. Elizabeth had discovered a shop in the outlet mall called "Hot Topic" that specialized in T-shirts of her favorite rock bands. We did not want to spend our educational trip at the mall, so we compromised with one hour there and one hour at the local Amish museum. The next day it was raining. We couldn't convince the children that it was charming to ride in an open buggy in a torrential downpour. We left for home early.

The Amish are also famous for their quilting skills, and in Lancaster I had bought a nine-patch heart quilt. Recently, however, I felt like an Amish quilt, walking around with estrogen patches stuck all over my stomach and rear. Once again it was hard to focus on anything else while undergoing my hormone treatments. As with every previous attempt, I felt placed in a state of limbo until the treatment cycle ended. At least this time there would be no agonized wait for a baby.

It was finally the right time to remove a piece of my uterus. It was the same doctor who had aspirated my cyst. I knew already that for this procedure all that was recommended was an Advil a half-hour before the biopsy.

The doctor informed me that I would be uncomfortable. First he would place all the equipment inside me, then pull down on my cervix. Just when I congratulated myself at having tolerated all of the pre-procedure pain, the doctor ordered the nurse to remove all of the equipment and announced that we would have to start all over again. "I can't find your uterus. I'll have to do a sonogram to figure out where it is," he explained. These were not the words I wanted to hear. If the doctor couldn't even find my uterus, how would he accurately remove a miniscule piece of uterine lining without puncturing an artery in the process?

"Ah, here is your uterus!" exclaimed the doctor as if he had just discovered America. "It was a little bit to the left, so that was why I couldn't find it. Now we can begin again." Once more the equipment was inserted. Then I felt the painful pinch of the needle in my uterus, and at last it was all over.

Two days later I was bleeding profusely. I was positive the doctor had nabbed tissue from the wrong place. I called the nurse in a panic. She informed me that by stopping the estrogen patches I had in effect gone off birth control pills and that my period had started.

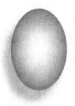

Blind Egg Date

As I became part of the donor egg process, I found my body image changing drastically. I felt like a 2002 model car on an assembly line and in need of all new parts. When I was "renovated" the shell would be the same, but the parts would be from younger donors.

Finally, after three months, the doctor took the time to read my uterine biopsy and give it his okay. Now I could progress on the donor egg waiting list. Around the same time, my forty-seventh birthday arrived. Forty-seven seemed as improbable for a bountiful womb as ninety for Sarah. I too would need a miracle.

It was now almost two years since I'd started IVF. My husband and I had spent all but six months of our marriage focused on my getting pregnant. Eventually, when this was over, we would have to find a new equilibrium with a focus on each other rather than on our baby quest. We did not want to become like those couples who banded together in the process of building an addition to their house, but floundered afterward because they had no other connection.

My brother, Mark, was a good model for me. After 9/11, he arrived at Ground Zero. He was not a fireman, EMT, or policeman. He just appeared and began clearing debris. Somehow he became "official" by joining the Red Cross. Subsequently, he remained in the Red Cross as a relief worker at disaster sites. He had no regrets about sitting back and becoming a spectator to his own life.

Every week, after attending a women's memoir-writing group, I would browse in the nearby antique mall. Each time, after seeing hundreds of items on all three floors of the building, my eyes would come to rest on the same two paintings. One was of a mother bedecked with roses, patiently sitting in a chair. Her two blonde daughters beamed as they brought her a birthday cake strewn with matching flowers. The other painting was of a mother proudly displaying her newborn baby. The first of these paintings always put me in mind of my own two blonde daughters. Would I ever have a similar connection to the second picture?

The old woman who owned the painting booth greeted me enthusiastically each week. I told her that I came to her after my memoir-writing group. I confided in her that I liked to stare at the painting with the newborn baby.

"I love that painting also. What do you like about it?"

"When I look at that portrait I think maybe one day I'll have a baby too. You see I'm trying to get pregnant. I'm in a second marriage, and I'm too old now. I'm using in vitro fertilization."

"Oh, there's a girl downstairs who did that for years. Every day I would see her come through the door crying. But it finally worked. She has a beautiful girl," explained the dealer. "You should meet her," she added.

The next week, when I reappeared at the booth, the dealer began waving a ticket in my face. "Here's a free entry to a downtown antique show. The girl I told you about is there today. She runs the Greek statue booth. Just look for the statues and tell her I sent you," she said.

Well, why not? In any case I'd get free admittance to the antique fair. I hopped the subway and found the show. There was only one booth with lithe, white headless Greek statues. I waited until the booth was empty of customers and screwed up my courage.

"Hello. This is going to sound a little bizarre. I'm not here about a statue. You see I met the older woman who sells artwork in your antiques building, and she told me about you. I'm trying to get pregnant with IVF," I explained hesitantly.

"Let's go get a cup of coffee," the woman replied warmly. She wore a long, flowing gown that matched the ancient Greece motif.

She left her co-worker in charge of the booth. We sat down in the café section amidst the antique Persian rugs. Immediately I launched into my IVF spiel. Then it was her turn.

"Well, let me tell you my story. I tried three times. Nothing happened the first two times, but I froze some eggs. The third time I thawed the eggs and got pregnant with my daughter." Then she gave me her advice. "Close the door behind you and move forward. It's time for something else. Go the donor egg route and don't look back."

Unlike me, she had never been told that her odds were low. She started IVF trials at forty-one and became pregnant at forty-two. Afterward she learned that, at age forty-two with a frozen egg, her chances had been one percent. If she'd known the tiny odds, she said, she'd never have even tried IVF. She felt I was lucky to know my chances were miniscule and that I should definitely detour onto the donor egg path.

I gave her a big hug and thanked her for being so helpful. I told her that I hoped one day I'd find her again in the Greek statue booth and have a baby to show her.

Unfortunately, her words did not have the desired effect. Her example did not motivate me to want a donor egg—just the opposite. I'd finally found a bona fide mother who had beat the odds. If she could have a baby with a one percent chance of success, then why couldn't I?

Priscilla was the Greek tragedy specialist of my women's writing group. She taught ancient Greek literature by night and attended our memoir group by day. That night, for the first time, Priscilla called me.

"Victoria, I'm about to go into class. I only have a moment but I have an answer to your project."

"What project?"

"Your baby project you've been writing about. I found you an egg," said Priscilla.

"An egg! From where?" I asked.

"It's my friend Lisa. She wants to give you her egg."

"Why?" I asked suspiciously.

"Well, she's getting a divorce and she needs the money. She wants me to tell you she was a champion swimmer. She's a little heavy now, but as a child she won awards. I also know she's a great shopper. She has a real flair for color," elaborated Priscilla.

Then came my million-dollar question, "Is she smart?"

"Well, she dropped out of school, but you can talk great politics with her."

"Do you think she'll want to visit the baby?" I asked.

"I don't know. Her own two children heard her talking about the eggs and want to know if they'll have a baby brother or sister. It was kind of weird. I have to go. But it's all set. We'll meet for lunch next week after our writers' group. Bye!"

It must have had something to do with Greece. When I was with the Greek statues, I was told "go donor." Now the Greek classics professor was going to give me her friend's egg.

Preparing for the encounter was like getting ready for a blind date. Should I wear my "dating clothes" far in the back of the closet? Sometimes they still came out for a Saturday night with Gabriel. However, I thought a conservative appearance would be best. I didn't want to wear anything revealing and look like the mom from *Desperate Housewives*, but I also didn't want to appear too frumpy.

The next week, in my writing group, I looked at my watch frequently. Soon Priscilla and I would meet Lisa in Au Bon Pain. I told Priscilla I needed to put on lipstick and brush my hair before we left. Priscilla said, "Don't worry. If it doesn't go well, I can always find you another egg." I thanked her for being a matchmaker.

Priscilla and I arrived at the café first. We pulled three chairs around the table for two. Lisa made her grand entrance. She wore big, dark movie star glasses and dramatically swung them over her forehead to reveal pretty green eyes. As Priscilla had mentioned, Lisa's svelte swimming days were a thing of the past. When Lisa returned with her tray, she spilled soup all over her lap. I reassured her that I often do the same thing. We passed around photos of our children. Lisa said her children used to model. She guaranteed me that she was very fertile and her eggs would work. However, we would have to hurry because in three months she would be thirty-five and too old to give her eggs. Chivalrously, Lisa held the swinging garbage top open while I emptied my lunch tray. She asked if I would have to check with my husband before I could commit to buying her eggs. Then, as if to confirm the success of our rendezvous, Lisa asked for my phone number and gave me hers. I told her she was very nice and that I had a good time. There was no kiss, but a goodbye hug.

I thanked Priscilla for her help. I wondered if Priscilla also knew that I wouldn't use Lisa's eggs. Lisa was too close to thirty-five and the odds of success were too slim. Also, I didn't want to have Lisa and her children ringing the bell to visit the baby. I was already dealing with my ex-husband's visitations with Lisette and Elizabeth. Would I have run the risk if Lisa had been a gorgeous genius? I don't know.

Yet another member from my memoir-writing group approached me about an egg possibility. The youngest member, who had been writing about life as a "twenty-something," was moving away. After her final meeting, we went to a pub for farewell drinks and hors d'oeuvres. As I was leaving the tavern with two other fellow writers, the youngest member ran to catch up with us.

"Victoria," she panted, "I have to tell you something."

"What?"

"I've thought about this carefully and talked to my mother. I'd like to give you one of my eggs. I'll do it before we move."

"Really?"

"Yes. I come from good stock. We have lots of doctors in my family, and I'd like you to have my egg."

"Well, that's very nice of you. I'll take your number."

I did not plan to call her. It was thoughtful of her to be inspired to offer me an egg as her goodbye gift, but I still wanted an anonymous donor. She didn't already have children that might visit their "half-sibling" like the other prospective donor, but she and her mother might still elect to see their family descendant and check out the continuation of their "good stock."

Chapter Five

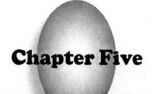

Last Roll of the Eggs

Hustling to Start–November 2004

After my blind date with Lisa, I called the donor egg nurse to check on my waitlist status.

"I have to be honest," she said. "We like to think it's moving quickly but it's really taking close to a year."

"If I want to, could I try again with my own egg in the meantime? I'm sure other people do that."

"Not really. We are the last stop for patients. If you try with your own egg you'll have to come off the donor egg waitlist," explained the nurse.

Not being one to take no for an answer, I called the other institution, the second I had tried. The nurse there said I could try with my own egg and be on their egg waitlist too at the same time.

I decided to burn the candle at both ends. I would stay on my original hospital's donor waitlist, which meant that I still had seven months of waiting left. At the same time I would try with my own egg at the second institution, without telling the first. As long as my donor egg didn't come early, it should all work out.

The problem was to convince Gabriel. I had already promised we would do a donor egg. Well, I would still try with a donor egg, but first I would just discreetly throw in another ten-thousand-dollar try with my own egg. If it had worked for the dealer in Greek antiquities, it could work for me.

"Gabriel, I called to check on our donor egg wait."

"That's great! What did they say?"

"The nurse says it's really taking a year no matter what anyone else says. That means it will still be months," I explained.

"Maybe it will go faster," said Gabriel.

"I told you if donor egg doesn't work, I want to try my egg again. But it's taking too long. By the time we try donor I may be too old and it will fail and it will be too late to try again for mine."

"Victoria, it's crazy to try your own egg again. It's just throwing away money. You already have two children of your own. Now I want one too," said Gabriel.

"My first choice is to try with my eggs again. I've already compromised by agreeing to a donor. I just want to try my eggs in the meantime."

There was silence on the phone line. Clearly we were locked in our own viewpoints and hurts and were temporarily immobilized.

The following day Gabriel said okay, I could try my eggs while we waited for the donor.

I felt very fortunate. Not all husbands would agree to five IVF trials with so little odds and so much cost. Of course, it was easier for him to be understanding because I had also committed to the donor egg road. And also he must have realized that I needed to go through all these failed IVF attempts with my own egg in order to be more ready to accept a donor egg.

Time did not stop for my egg trials. It was Christmas again, two years after my first IVF attempt. The title of the television Christmas special was *A Home for the Holidays* and it featured the adoption of children. I decided to watch it, hoping to be inspired in case I used a donor egg. There were testimonials of parents and children who had become a family after last year's TV special. The parents had picked the children from the broadcast and voilà!—they had become an instant family. I felt a flood of altruism as I thought of rescuing a child from an orphanage.

Then I tried to transfer this feeling to using a donor egg. It didn't work. I was not saving anyone by extracting someone's egg. The egg would become a monthly menstrual flow, not an abandoned baby desperate to have a home for the holidays.

A few days after the program, it was time for a flight to Florida.

Gabriel, Elizabeth, Lisette, and I traveled together. Elizabeth had her iPod, and Lisette had a portable DVD player with the new movie *Princess Diaries 2*. Gabriel slept, and I read. The latest electronic gadgets had made traveling pleasant rather than a test of parental endurance.

The plan was to arrive at my parents' house. Next we would call my ex-husband, Pierre, to come and get the kids. Gabriel and I would have four days without children. There were some benefits to divorce. I had half of Christmas vacation, two weeks in August, and a smattering of weekends during the year to utilize my ex as a baby-sitting service. During that time Gabriel and I strived to reclaim our dating life before we became a readymade family.

Gabriel was standing by the circling rubber conveyor belt waiting for the last piece of luggage. The children and I guarded a clump of already claimed suitcases. Then Pierre sauntered over.

"Hello, girls! I just happen to be here picking up my sister. Hello, Victoria. I didn't know I'd be here but my sister's flight got diverted from West Palm to Fort Lauderdale. I might as well take the girls now."

"Can you fit their luggage and your sister's and her kid's suitcases in the car?"

"Well, maybe not," admitted Pierre.

"I'm not going without my suitcase!" exclaimed Elizabeth.

"I'm not either," added Lisette.

"So, maybe then you can get the kids afterward as planned," I suggested. I was relieved, because my parents had wanted to see the children for a little while before they went off to celebrate Christmas with Pierre's family.

"I'll be right back," I said.

I ran over to forewarn Gabriel that Pierre was in the airport. The two had never met; normally I just transferred the girls to Pierre at our local diner.

Gabriel now came over with the last suitcase. "Hello."

Pierre extended his hand and said, "I'm so glad to meet you. It's a real pleasure."

Pierre wanted to appear charming even to my new husband. Unfortunately, the allure was only at a superficial level.

The next morning, ironically enough, Gabriel and I enjoyed our childlessness. We leisurely read the *New York Times*. This week the magazine section focused on people who had died in 2004, and I wanted to read about Marlon Brando.

Gabriel gulped his coffee, I sipped my tea, and then I saw a headline proclaiming "Donor Egg." This was not an invitation to donate eggs, but a full-page ad offering to sell them. Over a hundred donors were available, many of them at the Ph.D. level. There was no waitlist and a listed website.

I immediately asked Gabriel to plug in his laptop and surfed the web to the appropriate site. Here was a full-fledged egg donor matchmaking service! There were undergraduates, law and psychology graduate students, a doctoral candidate in molecular biology, and one promising medical student. The heights and weights, eye and hair color, educational level, and hobbies of each potential donor were listed. There also was an icon to click on the childhood photo of the donor. The first person I clicked, the medical student, had an adorable toddler picture, blonde hair adorned with a headband, and she was wearing a party dress. I soon realized, however, that every subsequent donor I clicked on used the identical photo!

I decided it was time to call the toll-free number. Gabriel was on the other extension. Immediately we were connected to the "intake nurse."

"Hi! I'm Victoria. I'm interested in knowing how your egg donor program works."

"Well, it's very simple. I can connect you with the registration department. We can register you over the phone and then you'll officially become one of our patients," explained the nurse.

"I have a question. How come every donor online has the same baby picture?"

"Oh, that's easy to explain. You see, that was a sample photo. Once you register and pay the five hundred and fifty dollars to become a patient, you'll get a computer ID number. Then you can download each official picture of the donor."

"Now it says in your ad that it takes only one day to come to your clinic for the egg. I live out of state. How do you do everything in one day?" I asked.

"You find a doctor to follow you where you live. You just come to have the egg transferred and your husband comes with his sperm."

Gabriel asked, "Are you affiliated with a hospital?"

The nurse answered, "I'm not sure."

Then I asked, "How much does it cost?"

"It normally costs twenty-five to thirty thousand dollars. However, you can split the eggs with someone else for cost reduction."

Gabriel wondered, "Are all the donors available for shared eggs?"

"Now, that is a good question. Only the best ones can supply two recipients at once. We can send you a list of our prized donors that are available for a shared cycle."

Gabriel then asked, "Are all donors available immediately?"

"No. You may have to wait if someone is in the middle of donating to someone else. All of our girls agree to donate three to nine times."

Now this was beginning to sound like a "puppy mill." When I bought my Shetland Sheepdog, I spoke with various dog breeders. They all warned against buying from a puppy mill where a few female dogs are used repeatedly to breed the puppies. In my head I calculated that if I used an egg producer who shared donations nine times, my own baby could have seventeen half-siblings, maybe more if the births resulted in twins or triplets.

We thanked the nurse and told her we'd think about it. She promised to mail us a list of the prime egg breeders. She also gave us the phone number of their financial department.

I liked the idea of being able to choose the egg myself rather than waiting a year for my current hospital to choose an egg for me. I also was happy with the high educational level of the donors. Gabriel thought it sounded like a purely moneymaking enterprise. He didn't believe it was good medical practice to have a third party monitor me and then for their facility to see me only once. He also didn't like that the nurse wasn't sure if there was an affiliated hospital. What if I had an emergency while the donor egg was being transferred into me?

Putting aside for the time being the idea of handpicking a donor egg, I refocused on my own egg cycle in the hope that it would work. As things turned out, I got my period early, right after I returned from Florida. I spoke with the doctor on call, and he confirmed that I should come in the following day.

The next morning, I rode the train to the hospital again. Right after my blood was drawn, I was directed to billing, the open area adjacent to the blood-drawing section. Here the financial clerks sat like bank tellers behind glass windows with a slot for sliding payments.

"We need your payment right away. We need one check for twelve thousand dollars and the second for the eight-hundred-dollar anesthesia bill."

"I don't have the checks today."

"Sorry, you have to pay to proceed."

"I'm good for the money. I paid the last two times. Can I bring in the money another day?"

"Tomorrow at the latest."

Now I was allowed to have my sonogram. It looked good. If my blood levels were also acceptable, I could start hormones that night. I decided to fill the prescription just in case. I called Gabriel so he could tell the local pharmacy we'd be picking up the medication later.

The nurse proudly showed me their latest gadget—a "pen" applicator for Follistim I'd be injecting. When the pen cap was depressed, a needle would appear and the medicine would be shot into my stomach. It reminded me of one of those trick spy inventions that you'd see on a tour of the FBI.

My husband called back. No pharmacy could obtain the Follistim by tonight. I'd have to go to the hospital pharmacy. My husband gave me the phone number to acquire insurance preauthorization from a hospital representative, but I couldn't get through to her. I decided to pay the pharmacy for just two of my ten required cartridges. How much could two vials of Follistim cost?

"That will be one thousand dollars," said the cashier.

"One thousand dollars!"

"That's right." I needed the medication, so I gave her my credit card. Then I sprinted back to the building with the office of the drug insurance coordinator. I asked to speak with the woman who handled drug approvals.

"Hi! I've been trying to reach you by phone," I panted.

Reluctantly she agreed to call in my approval.

Then I ran back to the pharmacy and got on the long line again. I told the cashier I now had approval. She checked, confirmed, and was nice enough to credit my card with the one thousand dollars.

Three and a half hours after my arrival at the hospital, I was all set. I had my medication for the evening, my pen gadget, and my thousand-dollar refund. Now I could go home on the train. This was the most pressured startup I'd had yet.

As if obtaining my medication had not seemed enough of a challenge, now I had to face telling the children I was trying again. I was dreading the prospect—they probably thought I'd given up by now. I decided to delay the confession as long as possible. The next time I went back to the hospital, I told them that Gabriel would have to drive them to school the next day because I had a doctor's appointment. They said nothing, and I was not yet forced to explain.

I tried the same approach the eve of my day-five blood-drawing. When I took Lisette aside privately and told her that I had another doctor's appointment in the morning, she said nothing. Elizabeth, however, who had recently turned fourteen, demanded: "Why?"

"I'm trying to have a baby again."

"Mom, forget it! Why don't you stop by now! This is ridiculous! You'll *never* have a baby."

I hadn't expected anything different from my teenager, but I fondly remembered a spring day six years earlier, when Elizabeth was eight. She had eagerly saved forty dollars from her holiday and birthday gifts and was excited about a carnival that had come to our hometown.

Elizabeth walked the perimeter of the fair, with all her savings in hand. She wasn't lured by the rides; instead, she went to the game booths that lined the edge of the fairgrounds. She stopped in front of one prize: a blonde-haired, green-eyed porcelain doll that wore a Victorian dress.

To win that doll, Elizabeth needed to roll balls down a wooden ramp. The balls must land in numbers that totaled very low or very high. Any in-between sum meant you lost.

Elizabeth paid for her first game. She confidently let those balls fly down the runway. Unfortunately, they did not land in a winning way. After a few more rounds of losing, I warned her, "Elizabeth, you should stop now."

"I want to keep going."

"Elizabeth, the odds are overwhelming that you're going to lose.

Only a few of those spaces will give you the right total. There's no way you can win."

"I'll try harder."

"The doll isn't even worth it. They sell porcelain dolls in the supermarket."

"I want that one."

Elizabeth changed her strategy. She was positive the new approach would work. She rolled the balls all the way from the left side. Then she rolled them all the way from the right side. It didn't matter. She still walked away without her forty dollars and without her doll.

Recently, Lisette had started recreational basketball, and after some practice she'd become a decent player. The coach was pleased because she grabbed the ball from her opponents during practice and made some baskets. The fact that she was one of the shortest team members didn't matter in sixth-grade basketball. Soon I had to explain to her that I might not be able to take her to all of her games because I might have conflicting doctor's appointments. In that case she would have to carpool.

"How come you have doctor appointments?" she asked.

"Well, you see, I'm trying to have a baby again."

"Don't come to any of my games! I don't want a pregnant mother sitting there. You're almost forty-seven. None of the other mothers have babies."

"Lisette, I'm not going to look pregnant yet. I won't show during your entire season. No one would notice."

"I don't care!"

Gabriel was disappointed that the children didn't want another brother or sister. In fact, Lisette wanted Gabriel to spend more time with her. She resented his work schedule and let him know it by being angry with him. Gabriel felt angry and withdrew. He somehow expected the children to confide in him like the kids on *Father Knows Best*. He also expected them to be quiet and well behaved. Since Gabriel was an only child, he didn't fight with his parents—he knew nothing about family screaming matches. In fact, he had been his parents' model child. He didn't break away from them for years and was not really ready for marriage until his parents were in their nineties.

The difficulties of step-parenting increased Gabriel's yearning for his own child. He was sure it would be easier to become the full-fledged father of a biological baby. He envisioned an obedient and supportive child, like himself.

On my day-eight sonogram, a stylish female doctor with French-tipped nails and frosty lipstick found six follicles.

"Six total? Oh no. That's the same as last January when I had a disastrous egg result—only one egg was decent."

I was crushed. What if I had no eggs for transfer this time? We'd have paid almost thirteen thousand dollars for my final effort, and there would be nothing at all to show for it, not even an embryo picture to add to my collection. Suddenly it seemed again the "eleventh hour." I was finding it harder and harder to hang on to my basic optimistic life philosophy that in the end, even at the last moment, everything would turn out right.

At times like these I often thought about the dark time when my first marriage dissolved. I had found a letter to Pierre from his California lover. The letter made it clear they'd been intimate. But the worst part was when I read about her being pregnant. I had an immediate, terrifying free-falling sensation. It was the same feeling I had had when Elizabeth, Lisette, and I crashed in the elevator of our Long Island apartment. The elevator had lost traction and fell from the fourth floor to below basement level. We screamed as the elevator hurled through space. Then we screamed some more because it was Labor Day and no one was around. Finally the building super heard us and pulled us out.

When I found other letters from Pierre's mistress, I realized that she'd miscarried their baby. There was at least some relief: to me and to the girls the worst betrayal would have been if he'd had a secret son somewhere. Pierre still wanted to stay married but demanded the right to mistresses. I responded by divorcing him three months later.

The breakup cost me my belief in simple happy endings. Eventually, though, I developed a conviction that without my first marriage I wouldn't have been the mother of Elizabeth and Lisette, and that without my divorce I wouldn't have met Gabriel. In the end everything did right itself.

By now my five IVF trials were taking a bodily toll: the increased hormones on the IVF trials frequently made me moody, and I was gaining weight too.

One Sunday when Lisette was at a birthday party, Gabriel was helping his parents, and I was planning to relax, Elizabeth emerged from her inner sanctum to demand that I take her to lunch. We ate at the local deli. Then, without explanation, she said we had to stop at a particular store. She would direct me there: it was really close, she promised. Thirty-five minutes later, we arrived at a thrift store called Second Hand Rose.

"This is an emergency," Elizabeth informed the salesman. "I need a record player right away."

"You mean the old kind that plays records?"

"Yes. The one that plays 'veneel,'" elaborated Elizabeth with her strange, decade-later interpretation of *vinyl*.

"Why do you need a record player?" inquired the clerk.

"Because I have to play music from the nineties. My favorites are only on records."

After all this, the man said, "We don't have any Victrolas. Besides, even if we did you'll never find the needles for them anyway. But you can try antique shops if you want."

We left the thrift shop.

Elizabeth said, "Okay, Mom, now you can take me to the antique shops. Will you pay for the record player? Also the records? I found some on eBay."

"No! I won't pay one cent for a record player or a record. I'm not going to spend my Sunday running around looking for a record player. You can make your own calls to stores and use your own money," I shouted in the street.

"Other mothers buy their children things."

"I buy you things too, but not this. You have an allowance."

"Thanks a lot, Mom."

Afterward it occurred to me that maybe I had been affected by all the hormones I was taking. Normally I would have waited to yell until we got home or at least were in the car with the windows closed. I was furious with Elizabeth.

That same day, after Lisette returned from her party, she spent the evening watching TV and instant-messaging her friends. At 9:45

p.m. she suddenly informed me that she had a science test the next day and asked me to quiz her on the material. She hadn't studied and didn't know a single item. Then she showed me the topics for an upcoming test about ancient Egypt.

"Lisette! Why are you watching TV and on the computer if you haven't studied a thing? It's almost ten o'clock. Your priorities are all messed up!" I screamed.

This time I felt rage, not just anger, as if I had metamorphosed into the Wicked Witch of the West. I knew that the hormones were working.

At least I was approaching the end of the last of my "own egg" trials. I was back in the hospital for my day-eleven blood and sonogram. My follicles had increased to nine.

The outgoing, loquacious physician confided, "I'm sorry you had to come again when you were just here yesterday. It's that darn doctor. She sends people every day for blood work. She kept that practice from the hospital where she used to work. Unfortunately, I work Thursdays and she works Wednesdays. I always have a full caseload from her. We always joke about who will have to work the day after her."

"What hospital did she used to work at?" I asked.

Of course it was my first institution—the one where I had had to traipse constantly into the city and wait forever.

The physician then told me, "The docs love to work the day after my shift. There is no one to see. I only make the patients come every three or four days."

"When will my eggs come out?" I asked.

"I'll be deciding this afternoon. If you have a tendency for overcooked eggs, we'll give you the hCG tonight, and your eggs will be out two days afterward. If your eggs tend to be undercooked, I'll wait until tomorrow for the hCG."

My hCG was that night. I guess I tend toward overdone eggs, and they needed to stop them before they became scrambled and fragmented.

Gabriel and I drove in for our respective retrievals—his sperm and my eggs. Gabriel was called almost immediately for sperm deposit. I was reading magazine articles in the upper mezzanine waiting area. In fact I almost finished the entire magazine. I wondered if Gabriel was having difficulty. Maybe they would ask me to help him.

Finally he emerged from a nearby office.

"I can't believe they used a movie trailer."

"What do you mean?"

"You know. I mean the kind of trailer you see before the real movie begins at the theater. Here there was no movie. Just the same clip playing over and over."

"Are you sure?"

"I tried everything. I put it on Video 1 and Video 2. No matter what, it just showed the same scene over and over again."

"What was the scene?"

"Oh, nothing," he replied evasively.

"Come on. I want to know."

"Well, it was a woman having oral sex with a man. Maybe they stopped supplying the video selection because the men were stealing the movies."

Now, on our fifth attempt, Gabriel sounded as jaded as the man who'd complained that the porn flicks were from the eighties. I was pleased that nine eggs were retrieved.

That night I felt well enough to go out to eat. Gabriel, Lisette, and I went to an Indian restaurant. Elizabeth was at a friend's house. I ordered a glass of white Zinfandel. It would be my last Saturday night glass of wine for a while. Once the eggs went back, I would refrain from all booze.

I held up a glass and proposed a toast. "To our new baby!"

I clicked my glass with Gabriel's. Lisette pulled her glass back.

"I have my own toast to make. I hope there's no baby!"

Gabriel was horrified. He wanted the children to be supportive and worried that if the baby ever materialized, Elizabeth and Lisette would treat it like Harry Potter at the Dursleys.

Our recently minted family was undergoing other tensions too. Once, when we were in the car together, Gabriel had talked about how meaningful it had been to his mother when Gabriel had taken her with him to temple. To which Elizabeth proclaimed, "Judaism just doesn't do very much for me."

"What does that mean?" asked Gabriel.

"It's nothing against Judaism. I just don't care much for any religion."

"What about your bat mitzvah?"

"I liked the party. It was fun."

Lisette did not make things any easier. When Gabriel crawled into our bed at night, he'd sometimes find popcorn under his blanket and pillow. "Who did this?" Gabriel asked.

"I'm sure it was Lisette," I answered.

"What was she doing in our bed? She doesn't belong here. She has her own bed. She's too big to sit in ours."

"She just likes to watch TV here."

Lisette further aggravated him when she left her snack plates around the house and ran off with his towel after showering in our bathroom.

"What's the matter with your kids?" Gabriel would turn on me. "You didn't discipline them right. You should have started at an earlier age."

"You can tell them not to do stuff."

"They don't listen to me."

"They don't always listen to either of us."

"I can't live like this anymore. I can't take it. I can't spend the rest of my life like this."

"Are you saying you want a divorce?"

"I'm just saying I can't take it."

"Gabriel, you'd better be sure you want all of us. I'm not having a baby so you can divorce me."

At times like these I thought of Star's question, "How's the marriage doing?" We didn't just have the stress of IVF. We were also trying to integrate a new stepfather into our family life, with me caught in the middle.

The day after our meal at the Indian restaurant came a call that only four of my eggs had fertilized. Then one hour before I took the train for my egg transfer, the phone rang. It was the nurse from my hospital. I panicked. They had never called me at an unscheduled time. They wanted to stop me from coming! There must not be anything to put back.

"Can you come later today? In the end only two of you had eggs that made it for transfer. We want to switch you near the other person's procedure."

I said, "Of course I'll change. I was scared you were canceling my transfer."

What a relief! I was sorry the other women had lost their eggs, but at least they weren't mine.

When I arrived at the hospital, I discovered that my own doctor would conduct my transfer. I hadn't seen him since we had first met almost a year earlier.

"Please sign your name here. We have three eggs to put back. You have one grade two and two grade three eggs. One of them divided six times, and the other two are a three and a four division."

"Last time I had much better eggs. These don't sound too good."

"Well, those eggs didn't get you pregnant last time," replied the doctor. I wasn't sure if he meant that as encouragement or not.

Once I was in the operating room, the embryologist asked me my name and social security number. She looked like Mother Goose with her white hair and wire-frame glasses. She was holding what looked like a shampoo bottle with a label on it.

"Are those my eggs?"

"No," she answered.

Three doctors were in the room—my male doctor, the slender female doctor, and the jovial anesthesiologist from my retrieval. My knees were draped over a shortened stirrup. My doctor was going to do a sonogram.

Then the female doctor said, "Don't move. There's something on your leg."

Something on my leg? Did the eggs roll out of the catheter?

"Was that the transfer already?" I asked.

"You're all done now," my doctor said.

"Good luck," the embryologist said. "If you become pregnant it will be from the six."

Then I was wheeled back to a corner of the recovery room. The curtains were drawn around me, and I was left with my legs up in the air. This was awful. Now I was waiting to become pregnant from embryos that might have been transferred to my leg. Also, from what the embryologist said, I had only one viable egg. The January hex still held. I began sobbing in solitude behind my curtains. This baby had no hope.

When I arrived home, I climbed in bed and put up my legs. I reached over to the drawer of the night table. Here were my prize score cards and embryo snapshots. No doubt about it. This was definitely the worst yield I'd had yet. When my husband wasn't looking, I sneaked out of bed to check the computer downstairs. My new embryo likenesses had not yet arrived. I wanted to see if they looked like flowers, or if they were bumpy and totally fragmented. My sense of hope was quickly being chipped away.

My mother called. "Hi, Victoria. I've been worried about you. How do you feel?"

"I feel okay, just a little cramping. I'm still upset about how bad my eggs were this time."

"Victoria, don't get your hopes up. The odds are overwhelmingly against you. I don't want you to be disappointed," my mother said.

"I know the odds are against me. I just told you my eggs are bad. Why try to dash whatever hope I have?"

I had decided at the outset that I would do the home pregnancy tests: That way I wouldn't be disgusted with myself when I did them even after making a firm resolution not to. Nonetheless, I was sick of the two-pink-line test and wanted to find a new one.

I went to two pharmacies and finally found a test that I hadn't tried before. There was an oval window that would always show a purple line, and a square window that would only display a line if there was a pregnancy. Best of all, the test came with a free gift, a pregnancy calendar. So now I would have yet another souvenir from prior attempts. Unfortunately, I had thrown out the failed pregnancy tests from all of my trials. If I had kept them, I could have created a three-dimensional collage to hang on the wall, titled "Missing."

Of course, the home pregnancy tests were negative, and then I went for the "real" blood test and decided to sit at home and wait for the phone to ring with the "real" result. This time I wanted a real voice with the news, not just a message left on my mobile phone.

I wished that my chances were better. My e-mail embryo photos were not promising. The six-cells egg was so bumpy it looked like a topographical map. The three-cells one had two prominent divisions that looked like pieces of stretched Silly Putty. What must have been the grade two egg was very smooth but had only four divisions. I was pretty certain that none of these embryos were viable. However, the nurse had told me that sometimes the worst-looking egg became a normal baby.

I would try and maintain hope. Maybe I had another James. Maybe this baby had an hCG too low to register on a home pregnancy test, but he was struggling to stay embedded in my womb.

The call was supposed to come between twelve and three p.m. At 2:45 there was still no ringing. By three I would dial them myself, I decided. The nurses probably saved the bearing of bad tidings for last. At 2:55 the phone rang.

"I am sorry," the nurse said. "I have not so good news. You are not pregnant. There is not even a possibility of something. Your hCG is a one."

She had tried to break the news to me in stages, but there had been no slow progression. As soon as she uttered, "I'm sorry," the message was clear.

Lisette burst into my room. "I was listening outside the door, Mom. I'm sorry it didn't work. Don't feel sad. I'll go tell Elizabeth." I watched Lisette run to Elizabeth's door. Lisette announced, "She's not pregnant" in a sorrowful tone, but then also gave a thumbs up sign to Elizabeth.

Elizabeth came over to me and said, "Mom, I'm sorry. You should stop now. You're just making yourself sad when it doesn't work. Five times is enough."

Gabriel was helping his parents when the no-pregnancy call came. I gave him the news over the phone. He was upset but not surprised.

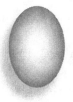

Do We Still Want a Baby?

I was picking up Lisette from school when the doctor called me on my cell phone for my phone consultation I was allowed after any failed trial. I told Lisette that she would have to wait outside the parked car. I didn't want her to overhear the egg donor discussion.

In fact, I wanted to check out with him a new procedure that Gabriel had been researching that I called "my Italian fantasy." Although I agreed with Elizabeth that five times was sufficient and that the route of my own egg was closed, I still needed to check this one last "miracle" possibility, which was known as a "cytoplasm transfer." For this technique the egg nucleus and cytoplasm were left intact. Instead the cytoplasm from a donor egg was inserted into the original egg to provide a boost. The donor cytoplasm would add the necessary rejuvenation for a more fertile, viable egg that could result in a pregnancy. On Google Gabriel had found research citations from four countries about cytoplasm transfer: Lebanon, Israel, Germany, and Italy. Germany, however, had a low success rate, and a number of women from fertility chat rooms reported their dissatisfaction with the pregnancy results there.

Italy sounded good to me. Gabriel and I could rent an Italian villa. We could eat pasta and drink fine wine (at least until my eggs were transferred back). We would create our own *Under the Tuscan Sun* movie. Meanwhile an Italian Dr. Frankenstein would be combining my egg with the cytoplasm from some young Gina Lollobrigida. The new creation would come to life from the spliced egg parts. There also was the possibility of a Frankenstein monster. Gabriel had read that there was a chance that the DNA from my nucleus, the donor's cytoplasm, and my husband's sperm could combine to create a deformed baby with too much genetic material. Still I wanted a baby enough that I thought I might risk it.

So I asked the doctor during our phone consultation whether I might not go to another country for a cytoplasm transfer or even a full nuclear transplant of my nucleus into someone else's egg. He said that yes, a nucleus transplant might correct the problem of aged eggs. However, there was no country performing this procedure anymore. I asked if there was a country where I could do it on the black market. He said no—there was nowhere to go. He told me I had two options—donor egg or my own egg with a new medication, micro-Lupron, to improve my egg quality. However, even if I took the micro-Lupron approach, my chances would still be in the single digits.

I still was a fighter, but there were no arenas left, not even in Italy. After the phone consultation, Lisette and I went to the Häagen-Dazs shop, one of our "mother-daughter" places. There we would usually have an ice cream cone while Lisette updated me on important events at school or at home. She wouldn't provide too many details, just an indirect but telling comment such as "I sit with Beth at lunch," which meant that her new acquaintance Beth was now her closest friend. This time we were celebrating her being cast as Wendy in *Peter Pan*, the lead role in the school play.

Lisette wanted to know what the doctor had said and why the trial hadn't worked. I told her that there was a way it could work with my egg and also part of a younger person's egg, but that doctors weren't allowed to do it anymore in the United States. Lisette wanted to know if the baby would still look like me. I told her that it would still be the part of my egg that should make the baby look like me. If I only used someone else's egg, on the other hand, the baby would not be from me in that way. Lisette told me, "Definitely don't do that."

It was becoming clear to me that if I used a donor egg, Lisette and Elizabeth would be even more negative about a new baby. It would be easier for me to tell them it had been my own egg. But I didn't want to lie, and if I kept a donor egg secret for years from Elizabeth and Lisette, they would be even more resentful. Could I wait until they grew attached to the baby before telling them? Would I tell my parents, relatives, and close friends? It wasn't the business of the whole community to know my egg source, but even if I resolved to lie to everyone else who asked about my egg, once Elizabeth knew she would tell all her friends, who would spread the word anyway.

And then there was the sibling rivalry that a demanding, bawling infant would provoke. After thirteen years, Lisette would lose her place as the "baby" of the family. Elizabeth would be less affected. But both might cause the baby emotional scarring by ignoring or relentlessly teasing it. They would have the ammunition to tell the baby that it was "a freak," conceived by a stranger's egg.

My hope was that once the child arrived, he or she would evoke love in everyone. Lisette and Elizabeth would feel kindness toward their new sibling. I would have the same attachment as if it was genetically mine. Gabriel, the only one with a genetic bond, would automatically feel attached.

Gabriel knew, though, that both children did not want a baby and that I still was ambivalent about a donor egg. "Victoria, I don't want to make everyone suffer. If all of you are really against the baby, we don't have to do anything."

"I didn't say I won't do a donor egg."

"I'm just going to be very depressed if I don't have a child of my own."

"I'll keep my promise, but I want to be more excited about someone else's egg."

I understood how Gabriel felt. If I had no children, I would have done anything to have one. I would have found it very difficult to conceive of a life without children. Gabriel had been very accepting of Elizabeth and Lisette and took them on as his own emotionally and financially. I felt I should want to provide him with a child no matter what the means.

I felt very sad. It was just that I could no longer maintain my "life is beautiful" outlook. Everything had not turned out okay in the end. I would not have my own wonderful baby with Gabriel. Before I had been convinced that somehow I was destined to succeed. Now I knew for sure that I was like every other woman. No lightning rod protected my womb against infertility.

I also spent time wondering at what point my eggs had turned "bad." My first IVF attempt, when I was the youngest, was my only pregnancy. Perhaps if we had tried during our engagement, I would have become pregnant. My friends Star and Jay had taken us to dinner when Gabriel and I became engaged. We confided to them that we wanted to have a baby together.

"You should start trying to have a baby immediately!" exclaimed Jay.

"Every day you wait, your chances decrease," said Star.

"But we're not even married yet!"

"It doesn't matter," said Jay.

"I don't want to be a pregnant bride."

"Because you're already forty-three your chances of becoming pregnant at all only keep falling, and that's just the reality," responded Jay.

Jay was nice enough not to say, "I told you so" after all of our failed attempts. But perhaps we should have listened to them. Maybe, if Gabriel and I had gone home after dinner and made unprotected love, I would have become pregnant. I would have been a blushing bride with my telltale belly, but at least I would have been a mother too.

Now, if I just focused on being able to have a baby, the donor egg felt like a good solution. But as soon as I thought about not being able to have another one of my own, it just felt tremendously painful. It was hard to fully address my feelings about a donor egg when I was still reeling from the loss of my own genetic pregnancy. Meanwhile Gabriel's enthusiasm about the donor egg with his sperm brought me into new conflict.

I decided to call Star again. "Star, Gabriel and I still don't agree about the donor egg."

"In the end, both of you may be unhappy."

"What do you mean?"

"After we had Jewel, Jay and I had one more IVF attempt. I miscarried. I wanted to try again. Jay refused. He said that I was getting too old at forty-two and that if we wanted a baby we should adopt. Then we'd definitely get one."

"So what happened?"

"I had been willing to adopt before we had Jewel. Once I had a child, I wasn't willing to adopt anymore. I only wanted our genes. Jay and I couldn't agree, so we did neither and did not get a sibling for Jewel. We were both unhappy."

I did not want both Gabriel and me to lose out. I would not renege on my donor egg promise to Gabriel. I just wanted to be happier about it.

Tammy, the woman who confessed that she had gotten pregnant with a donor egg, had told me about a donor egg group, so I decided to call its leader. She told me there was a group for women who were considering becoming donor egg mothers, but since it had already met twice, it would disrupt the group dynamics if I joined for the third meeting.

"What if I don't ask questions and don't hold them back?" I asked.

The leader, who was a psychologist, said no but that, in the meantime, I could meet with her individually. I told her that I really wanted to hear what other women thought about a donor egg, but I made an appointment anyway, since that was my only option.

When it was time for my appointment I went right into the office without having to wait, and I chose the comfortable armchair instead of the couch. I told the psychologist that I was on a donor egg waitlist, and I might be contacted anytime within the next four months. However, whenever I thought about a donor egg baby it just made me sad, because I associated it with the loss of my own biological child.

The psychologist told me I needed to separate those two issues. One issue was mourning for the loss of my biological child, and that would take time. The other issue was whether I really wanted to have a baby with a donor egg. I ought to decide that separately from my feelings of loss. Having a baby just to honor a verbal agreement with my husband and to make him happy that was not a good enough reason.

My decision, she said, might well be different from that of other women. Most donor egg candidates were older women with no children. They wanted a first child no matter what and had to decide between adoption and IVF with someone else's egg. The psychologist said that in my case I could be happy without another baby. I had to weigh how much I wanted a child with my new husband against all the sacrifices in lifestyle that having another child would entail. She also pointed out that even if I was in the group she was running, it might not be helpful for me, because I was facing choices different from everyone else's.

I told her that I wouldn't care about the sacrifices if it were my biological child. With a donor egg, I did think more about what I would give up. I could never just walk out of the house and leave the baby alone. Elizabeth could babysit other children now, and Lisette could be left alone for a few hours. I was just beginning to taste freedom. All that would be gone, as would all spontaneity in plans between Gabriel and me. We would have to arrange childcare before every outing. We might never have a child-free retirement or be able to travel around the world. Instead I might still be working to put my third child through college. I could even be dead by the time he or she graduated.

The psychologist recommended that my husband and I do some serious talking together. "What will you do when you get the phone call saying your donor egg is ready?" she asked. "You have to decide beforehand."

I told her it had been hard to focus on a donor egg because I had never really closed the door on using my own egg. However, now the door appeared closed (although I always liked to leave the possibility open for a new discovery).

I wanted to be ecstatic about having a baby—any baby. I hoped to feel joy and excitement when I got the donor egg phone call. I told her that if there was a group opening, I still wanted to attend. Even if other women's circumstances were different, they would also have to mourn the loss of their biological child—perhaps even more so if they never had one of their own. They too must transition to the happiness of having a baby, whatever the means. I didn't just want to hear how other women accepted a donor egg but also focus on my own internal process. I thanked the psychologist and said goodbye.

Meanwhile Elizabeth felt free to give me her own unsolicited advice. She asked, "Mom, you're not thinking about trying any more, are you?"

I responded, "I don't know."

"Mom, forget about having a baby. Also, stop writing about it already. It will be a boring book, anyway. The first part will be 'I tried to have a baby—it didn't work.' The next section will be 'I tried again, and it did not work.' The third and fourth parts will be 'I tried more times and did not succeed.' Then it will say 'I tried once more and still failed.'"

Elizabeth's final words of advice: "Make it up. Write as your ending—'I tried again and got pregnant.'"

So, even Elizabeth would give me the happy American movie ending. In truth, my efforts might result in the bleak, European version: all efforts leading to the existential truth of nothingness.

Soon afterward, Gabriel and I had our romantic Valentine's Day dinner. Both of us dressed up. I wore a skirt and panty hose rather than my winter "cheat" of boots with knee socks underneath. The setting was a castle—originally the home of a nineteenth-century robber baron. The tables for two were in rows. Each woman received a rose, and each man a small box of chocolates.

Gabriel and I held hands. We gazed into each other's eyes. We said "I love you" a number of times and exchanged cards and gifts. Then we got down to business—talking about the donor egg.

I reported to Gabriel what the group leader had told me. I said that I had to really want this baby. It wouldn't be right for me to have the baby just to please him and then not to be accepting of it.

Gabriel reiterated that we could decide to do nothing. Then he said once again that he would be really sad, because he wanted a child of his own.

I felt bad because Gabriel and I were not entirely in sync. I told him that I would proceed with the donor egg, but that I wanted to become more positive about it. There also was a larger issue. Given our obsession with overcoming all the obstacles in our baby quest, had we maybe forgotten to ask another question—whether we really still wanted it? As the process went on for more years, wasn't it possible we might change our minds? That we might feel too old or become satisfied with our family as it was, without any new additions?

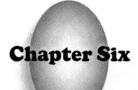

Chapter Six

Online Egg Mall

Shopaholic–February 2005

The psychologist running the donor egg recipient group had told me that her clients were not all obtaining their eggs from a hospital. Many preferred to find them from the internet. She wasn't making an endorsement, she said. It was just a suggestion.

The internet—I immediately thought of eBay! I knew all about eBay from my earlier search for silver lion pieces. I opened a Google search window and entered "eBay buy donor eggs." What came up was a spectacular eBay auction. A famous fashion photographer had arranged an auction for the eggs of eight beautiful models. Bidding was to start at fifteen thousand and could go as high as one hundred and fifty thousand. There was a lot of dispute; the photographer claimed to have had three children from three different spouses, and that only the last of his children had ended up beautiful but he treated them all the same anyway. Now other families could try to create gorgeous babies from the models' eggs. This auction, however, which was to have taken place in 1999, never happened—at least not on eBay. It was canceled and all future egg sales were prohibited. That was okay with me: buying a potential child off an auction block felt distasteful.

The auctions on eBay were closed for egg sale, but what about other internet sites? One evening I went back online and did not get off again until two a.m. There were a countless number of choices. California was the biggest egg mall of them all. First were the sites that catered to appearance and advertised "beautiful" egg donors. With a click of the mouse, you could find an array of headshots. All of the women looked like movie stars. Many of the photos were full-length pinup shots to accentuate the desirability of the body as well as the face. At one site I activated a video and watched a blonde, blue-eyed egg donor hopeful named Sunshine. She loved to work out to stay fit, she said, and to eat well. She aspired to be a famous actress. Most of these women had dropped out of college or else had never attended.

Other donor markets specialized in intelligence. These shops supplied Ivy League or high SAT-score eggs. Donors came from all around the country. One particular company was cited as the premier sales site for Ivy League donors. When I went on this site, I saw an "Urgent Notice!" They had been forced to shut down immediately. Donors and recipients in the middle of their cycles would have to fend for themselves. Records would not be released unless requested in writing. Something awful must have happened. Had their Ivy League donors really been bootleg eggs obtained from desperate, illegal aliens attempting to cross the border?

There also were "two-tier" egg stores. On these, an "extraordinary" or "exceptional" donor with a strong educational pedigree cost more than the "ordinary" donor—sort of like Saks versus Wal-Mart. Another mark of an extraordinary donor was someone who had successfully donated eggs before. Some donors even proclaimed their fertility by announcing that their eggs had produced twins or triplets. Just what I needed!

The California site also offered different degrees of contact between donor and recipient. The most open condition was one with an initial luncheon rendezvous. Under this arrangement, the donor could later become part of the "extended" family. There would be visits to the biological child and the exchange of correspondence and photos. I had long ago eliminated that possibility.

The next level of contact was one-sided. The recipient would know a lot about the donor, but to the donor she remained anonymous. At the third level, neither side knew much about the other party.

Besides donor egg sites, I found donor egg directories. They operated like hotel guides, with symbols for each level of amenity. A camera with the "PC" acronym meant that you had access to a photo from the donor's childhood. "PA" on the camera meant a photo from the donor's adult life. A donor egg facility with a "NO" or "X" sign offered no services.

Egg facilities came in three forms. Clinics provided both eggs and medical services; many also supplied a lot of information about the donor. Agencies acted as middlemen who matched donor and recipient but provided no medical care. An agency received a set fee or else a percentage of the donor's fee. Hospitals were the third type of egg boutique and seemed to operate in a similar manner. There was a waitlist of about a year. A cost-saving plan might allow for sharing eggs with another recipient, in which case costs of medication and medical procedures as well as the donor fee were all split. The price for having a donor all to yourself was almost doubled. At hospitals you saw no photos or SAT scores, and you never met the donor. The hospital called about a year after you signed up and assigned your egg donor. You had a right to refuse, but no right to choose. The hospital waitlist that I'd been on for almost a year worked in this manner.

Having at last surveyed the possibilities helped me. I was no longer sure if I wanted the hospital method anymore. I wanted to be an educated consumer, and I was in the "shop 'til you drop" mode. I continued my online window-shopping into the start of the next day. There were so many choices! Did I want the beautiful egg or the "egghead"? Better yet, why not the mix of looks and brains! Some of the donors could be ordered right away—by their first name or their assigned serial number. Slowly I put together a list of my top picks.

Then I lay awake in bed. Initially my shopping high kept me awake. Soon I began to have second thoughts. Did I really want to focus on breeding an "extraordinary" baby? Wasn't this just reverting to my old double standard of higher expectations for a donor baby than for my own? If I was ready to accept my own infant as flawed, then why should a donor baby have to be perfect?

I thought about the "sleeper" gene I might well have inherited from my great-grandmother Rivka. She had been my mother's paternal grandmother; she arrived from the old country as a teenager. There were many pictures of Rivka. The most distinctive show her at the beach with my mother, who was about eight. Rivka wore the old-fashioned bathing suit with the swimming trunks to the knees and the matching tank top. Despite the modest nature of these suits, Rivka's figure still stood out. She looked like a beached whale lying in the sand next to my mother. Her harsh, unsmiling face might have stopped a clock. Her personality was very fine—if you were a boy. My mother and aunt were treated like Cinderellas while the two male grandchildren were Prince Charmings. Rivka missed the old country. At age eighty-eight, she did a reverse commute from Ellis Island to Poland. Unfortunately, when she arrived everyone she had known was already dead. Nonetheless, she was taken in by a convent and died among the nuns at age ninety-five. Any one of my eggs could recreate Rivka. And with that kind of intolerance and insensitivity liable to surface in my own background, why worry about the perfect egg donor?

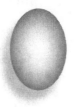

Egg McMuffin

Originally James had been due to be born the day of Elizabeth's bat mitzvah. When I spoke to the temple about changing her date, they had said all dates were taken, until finally they said we could have Christmas vacation. Elizabeth wasn't happy with her new day, but then James was never born, so we never switched the date.

Elizabeth had had other bat mitzvah woes. Her friend Melissa's bat mitzvah was the week before Elizabeth's, and three weeks before her party she'd gone with Melissa to pick up Melissa's bat mitzvah dress. It was the same as Elizabeth's outfit! Elizabeth cried in her room for the rest of the day.

Of course we altered Elizabeth's dress, by adding lace to the bottom. It looked like a new creation, and Elizabeth was happy.

An invitation in the mail caused the next bat mitzvah trauma. Elizabeth was one of the youngest in the class, so I'd thought there could be no more affairs after hers. Yet when she opened the invitation, she saw it was for the bar mitzvah of a boy in her school, the same day and time as hers! Elizabeth immediately took to her room sobbing; her bat mitzvah was becoming as complicated as a debutante's coming out party. This crisis also passed. Most of the boys went to the boy's bar mitzvah, and the girls to hers. Luckily her party predated the Sweet Sixteen stage when boys and girls would want to be together.

Now it was time to start again with Lisette. The original assigned date was a year and a half in advance, during the spring school vacation when most of her friends would be away. We went back to the synagogue for another date. There weren't any. However, at the last moment someone abandoned her day, and we got it. Everything was calm—until I realized the likely timing for my donor egg.

Most probably I would be called just in time to create a delivery date nearly identical with that of Lisette's bat mitzvah. If Lisette didn't want a pregnant mother at her basketball game, she definitely wouldn't want me pregnant at her bat mitzvah! Normally I was thin, but with Elizabeth I had gained forty pounds, and with Lisette sixty. If I kept up that pattern, I'd gain eighty pounds with a donor baby. Then I'd be waddling around the bat mitzvah evoking the essence of great-grand-mother Rivka. As I danced the Hora, I would go into labor.

Now I would have to act fast or wait almost nine months to make sure that I was no more than five months' pregnant at Lisette's bat mitzvah. I called my first hospital to see how I was doing on the wait-list. The egg donor coordinator looked me up in the computer.

She said, "In one month you'll have been on the waitlist for a year."

"Really? That's great! I calculated that I had a few more months to wait."

"Well, a year on the waitlist doesn't guarantee anything. You don't have a number stamped on your back."

"Is there a chance I'll be called soon?"

"Perhaps," she said.

"This is going to sound silly, but if my eggs don't go in soon I'm likely to deliver just in time for my daughter's bat mitzvah. I either need to start right away or else wait a while."

"Even if you get called with a donor, it could take months before implantation. We have to coordinate the menstrual cycles of three people—you, the other recipient, and the egg donor. But be assured, we're working hard on a good match for you."

I asked her more about the good match. I reiterated that I wanted someone bright. I told her that it wasn't essential but preferable if the donor looked like my children. My children had the recessive genes. Their coloring was similar to my grandmother, cousins, aunts, uncles, and nieces on my maternal side. The coordinator said they would be matching my own coloring. She also said they definitely wouldn't give me a blue-eyed donor. But I had a blue-eyed gene from my grand-mother, I told her. She said that didn't matter. I still didn't think the good match was in accordance with what I wanted. And they were taking over a year to match my eye and hair color.

If I wanted to make this happen I would have to speed things along. If I delayed another nine months, I'd be almost fifty when I delivered.

I began by window-shopping in the Magic Kingdom. We were spending four days in Disney World with the children. While other people gazed at the rides, I looked at the patrons. I studied the facial structures of the children and their respective parents. I noted what combinations of physical characteristics produced what types of children. I became my own genetic breeding expert. After Disney, we spent a few days with my parents.

My cousin Katie and her husband also were in Florida visiting Katie's mother, my aunt Dottie. Saturday night the adult cousins all went out to dinner. My parents watched Elizabeth and Lisette. I told Katie and Matthew that I was trying to find an egg donor quickly. I explained my hospital waitlist wouldn't come through in time, so I'd have to use the internet. They were amazed that donors were posted online. After dinner they offered to help us locate a donor. I told them if they found a good one, they could become the godparents.

We went to the library at my parents' clubhouse. My parents re-sided in one of those Florida communities that come with a built-in social scene centered around the clubhouse; theirs included a party room, dining room, card room, and spa. First we logged onto the site that Gabriel and I first saw over Christmas vacation, the place that advertised in the *New York Times Magazine*.

In fact I had already been in touch with this agency by cell phone while the children were waiting on a long line for a ride on Space Mountain in Disney World. The nurse told me that I could look at their donor base and pick a donor quickly but that some of their do-nors had a waitlist. I asked if it was the more educated ones who were in greatest demand. She explained that originally they had targeted their program for educational achievement, thinking there would be a rush for bright donors. However, recently they had extended their program to include adult photos rather than just baby pictures. The adult photos were not online, but you could travel to their office and view the photos onsite. This additional service had changed everything. Now customers preferred a good-looking donor to a smart one.

Katie, Matthew, Gabriel, and I looked at every donor profile on their website. We took turns sitting in the chair facing the computer and clicking the mouse. Once we got to the more detailed informational section, every donor we had picked from the profile highlights turned out to have something we didn't like about her. One was the carrier of a genetic disorder. Another's relatives had died from heart attacks at a young age. All of us were in good shape, and we avoided picking donors whose listed height and weight were in gross discrepancy. We also stayed away from women under five feet and over six feet tall. We were so picky, I probably wouldn't even have chosen myself.

Then we switched to the California sites that carried adult photos. Katie preferred the ones who looked like models. Maybe there was something to what the nurse had told me on the phone—once you saw a person, you picked differently. Significantly Gabriel even dismissed one because he said he never would have dated her.

One woman displayed herself in nothing but a Turkish towel carelessly draped across her lap, hands cupping her bare breasts. Her body proportions may have been perfect for a painting by Rubens, but needless to say she was not the pick that would make my cousins godparents. In fact no one was. I would have to continue my hunt after we returned home.

After we returned from Florida, I spent two days nonstop on the computer. I sat at the computer table in the basement with the dog in my lap. I was going back to work on the third day so I hoped for a quick success. My best hours were while the children were in school. The easiest sites to access had immediate entry, and other sites required a password, available by calling a phone number or registering online. I eliminated the sites that required an entry fee for an initial viewing. I also did not pay if they demanded money for a second viewing of the more detailed information such as donor essays and medical histories. Some questions were not critical anyway. For instance, on one site the donors had been asked if they believed in magic or slept with a stuffed animal.

The donor usually offered some statement about why they were donating eggs. Some were becoming mothers themselves and expected to be a second mother to the recipient's baby and become part of the recipient's family. They required a meeting with the recipient and expected to feel sympatico with the co-parent. One woman wanted to populate the world with her unusual eye color. Most women admitted that they needed the money, even as they claimed to be thrilled to be helping another couple conceive. In truth, I felt newfound respect for many of the donors.

The availability of donors was also listed. Some were ready to start immediately. Others were already "in cycle" with someone else. The more popular ones were currently in use and already reserved for their next two ovulatory cycles. A number of donors were traveling or studying abroad. However, if you paid their roundtrip airfare you could bring them over for an egg retrieval before flying them back to the wonders of Europe. A donor in France looked promising. I called the agent about her, but she told me the woman was not one of their premier donors, that the donor's father was an alcoholic and cocaine addict. I thanked the agent for her honesty.

Another agent told me that donors frequently used made-up first names for their internet listing to avoid being staked out by desperate, potential egg recipient parents who figured out their identities from first name, photo, and listed place of residence.

Among the women who listed their IQs were a number of very smart people. One woman who claimed her IQ was 156 had a grade point average of 2.0. Another woman said her IQ of 145 was based on a kindergarten test—probably naptime.

I decided to choose agencies that required documentation. For example, a donor would need to provide a transcript to document her 4.0 average or SAT results or a diploma to prove she actually had a college degree. After two days I finally found two acceptable candidates, one from the East coast and one from the West.

Both donors were attractive and had coloring that matched my children. The first donor, from New England, was brilliant. Her college entrance exam was almost perfect, her resumé phenomenal. She was already more accomplished than most of my friends double her age. Here at last was a bona fide intellectually gifted donor. In fact I was worried that she was too smart. After all, I wanted my child to be a "regular kid," and I wasn't sure if this donor egg child would be invited to any birthday parties.

The second donor discovery, from California, was studying a field that was academically difficult, so I figured she must be bright. Her college entrance exam scores also were high.

The complication was that neither donor lived near me. My original institution, where I remained on the donor egg waitlist, did not allow recipients to bring in their own donors, unless it was a close relation such as your sister. My second institution, which did allow it, required recipients not only to pay for a donor's travel expenses but also for a month's worth of meals and hotel accommodations as well as a subsidized companion. There was a cheaper route: to do the procedure at a facility near her. I could be monitored by my hospital, while she was followed by hers. At the proper moment my husband would fly out for sperm deposit, and three to five days later (depending on the development of the embryo) I would fly out for embryo transfer. All of these flights, of course, also cost money.

Another issue was the quality of the facility. Gabriel found a site from RESOLVE: The National Infertility Association with a link to the donor egg pregnancy rates reported to the Centers for Disease Control. A number of places did not cite their results or else reported success rates based on two or three egg donor transfers for an entire year. I began calling the facilities near each of my potential egg donors that listed decent pregnancy statistics. Many of the New England clinics near the first donor would not accept me—I was already too old! Their cutoff was forty-five. Finally I found an available office near the second donor. Everything would have to work perfectly for the baby to be transferred in time. At least there was a chance. I resolved to go with the second donor.

Next I investigated the legal questions. What laws would apply? The egg was coming from one state, the womb mother from another. The transfer would occur in the donor's home state, but the baby would be delivered in mine. I asked the donor's agent about California's laws. I wanted to make sure there were no provisions for joint custody between donor and recipient mother. I also wanted to be certain that the identity of the donor remained sealed. Otherwise it could become very complicated. If there were ever a dispute, we could end up in the tabloids as one of those sensationalist cases. The agent reassured me that California laws were tilted in favor of the recipient. She even had a lawyer call me to confirm that the baby would be one hundred percent mine.

It was hard to time my research project properly. Lisette came downstairs to the basement while I was printing photos of potential donors. She grabbed one and wanted to know what I was doing. Then she said, "Oh, I know. You're printing people who had babies. Look at them, Mom. They're in their twenties. No wonder they had a baby. You know you're too old." I did not disabuse her.

One of my long-standing diversions had been renting scary movies. In fact I was a bit of a horror movie aficionado. As a child, I had watched the *Creature Feature* and *Chiller Theatre*, and I especially liked vampire movies. Later I was drawn to movies such as *Nightmare on Elm Street* and *The Shining*.

Unfortunately, the DVD I rented in the midst of my computer egg quest was not conducive to my feeling more comfortable with my donor egg option. Entitled *Blessed,* it was about an infertile couple who went to have an IVF cycle at a sterile, sinister-looking facility where, unbeknownst to them, the doctors switched the husband's sperm for the seed of Satan himself. The woman gave birth to two daughters—beautiful angelic-appearing ones who later made the face rot off of a bratty boy.

This was not the best movie for me. What if my agency really kept the donor's fee and instead provided me with one from a homeless woman who was a secret subway sociopath who pushed commuters off the tracks and into the oncoming trains? I was vulnerable to this horror flick because I still had a feeling that any donor egg baby would be an "alien" implanted in my womb. I did not really think a satanic monster would emerge as in *Rosemary's Baby*. Still I had an unshakable conviction that this donor baby was "not me" and that I would not be able to love it as my own.

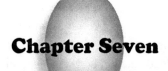

Chapter Seven

Disappearing Eggs

"Hava Nagila"—March 2005

The nurse at my newfound California facility told me that there were three initial steps. I needed to start birth control pills to suppress ovulation, have a phone consult with the California doctor, and have him conduct a physical exam for the egg donor and test her blood for sexually transmitted diseases (STDs). If my donor had a significant other, than he or she must also be evaluated for STDs.

The nurse asked the date of my last period. I was eight days post-period, I told her. This was going to be really close, she said—either I was starting birth control just in time or I had just missed. If I had missed, I might not finish the transfer in accordance with my time-table. She'd have to ask the doctor. In the meantime, I was told to fill the birth control prescription just in case.

Luckily I made it. I could go on the pill. The nurse cautioned me that the pills might not be effective—there was a chance I could become pregnant. After six months of trying on our own and five failed IVF attempts, I did not think there was much danger of my becoming pregnant. I'd take the risk!

Being prescribed birth control pills for IVF was a first, and I was somewhat anxious about their effect. In fact, I'd never taken them, and I knew a woman who was in the miniscule, serious birth control pill side-effect category. She'd started pills when her child was still an infant and had suffered a massive stroke while only in her twenties. Since then, she'd been unable to hold her own baby and required round-the-clock nursing care. I certainly hoped that wouldn't happen to me. At least I'd be on the pill for only a number of weeks.

My choice of donor made me feel good. I liked what she wrote in her profile. She seemed like a nice person as well as being smart and pretty. I was more involved in the donor egg process now that I had selected her myself. She would be the representative of my side of the family.

I had planned to be a detective, even if I went through my hospital donor egg program. This was my plan: when I went to the hospital for blood work, I would track whoever came in around the same time as me and identify all the women young enough to be my egg donor. I would nonchalantly strike up conversations in the waiting room in an effort to discover if they were donating eggs. I would try to learn as much information about them as possible, without becoming an "egg stalker mom." If my sleuthing was successful, I would know something about my egg donor.

None of this was necessary with my newly discovered donor. I already knew a lot about her. I did not want to meet her in the clinic waiting room. I could not risk her identifying me and coming to visit her baby. I was glad to have information about her life and her physical appearance. But sometimes too much knowledge can be a dangerous thing. Already, I could picture her having sex with Gabriel. She was almost twenty years younger than I was and probably in much better shape. Gabriel reassured me that he did not want to have sex with her. They were just inserting his sperm into her egg at the lab. I tried to think of it as comparable to when I deposit my clothing in the Salvation Army drop-off box. The person who would wear my clothes was not connected to me. Only in this situation I was the charity case for my egg donor.

I had my phone consult with the California physician. He told me I could have the embryos genetically tested to make sure they had no defects. I also had the option to pick the gender of my baby.

When Gabriel returned home from work, I relayed my conversation with the doctor. We were sitting in our dining room with the lace curtains and opaque liners that prevent people from looking inside as they walk by our house. Gabriel perked up when I told him we could choose the sex of our child.

"Oh, really," he said.

"I told the doctor it wouldn't be necessary."

"Why would you tell him that?"

I don't know why I was surprised that Gabriel was interested in sex selection, that he wanted a boy above all. In that way he could create the ninth link of the unbroken chain of male descendants from his famous ancestor.

Originally, before I had children, I wanted a girl and a boy. When Elizabeth was born, I had known beforehand that she was a girl. Her Alpha-fetoprotein screening had proved a false positive for spinal bifida, a congenital disorder with incomplete closing of the spinal cord. I waited anxiously for the amniocentesis. The amnio was normal, and in the process I learned that Elizabeth was a girl.

With Lisette, I had wanted to be surprised. I instructed the doctor not to tell me the sex after my amniocentesis, even though everyone else in the office knew. Whenever I went for checkups, the nurses referred to the baby as "he." I was positive that Lisette was a boy. I bought cute blue outfits and decorated her room with pictures of boys.

I experienced long labors with both Elizabeth and Lisette. Both times I didn't dilate much until the end, when it was too late for an epidural. With Elizabeth I was high on Stadol and felt as though I was riding a Ferris wheel in an amusement park. With Lisette I was in agonizing pain and screamed so loudly that the nurses said I was freaking out the teenage mother across the hall. When I finally began to dilate, the nurse said, "Let's get her going," then clapped her hand over her mouth and said, "Oops." Only at that point did I know I would have another daughter.

I did not care about the sex this time. I also would be glad to have my first son, but Elizabeth and Lisette were so wonderful that I had no problem envisioning another girl.

Gabriel said, "We are orchestrating everything else. Why not choose the sex too?"

I thought choosing the sex might be going too far. Maybe it was fate for a certain baby to be born. If the doctor picked the embryo, then it changed destiny. Perhaps he would prevent the birth of the child who was supposed to discover the cure for cancer. Gabriel reluctantly agreed not to choose the sex—primarily because it would have cost more money.

Meanwhile, now that I was going forward with the donor egg, I decided that I really must become more accepting of my choice. Again, I hoped to become part of a group with other recipients in the same situation. I asked my second hospital if I could meet their psychologist for an individual counseling session and then attend a one-session group. They agreed.

When it came time to meet with the psychologist, I told her that I was still sad about my recent failed IVF attempt. The counselor said she could help me to accept a donor egg baby, and I felt a strong connection to her right away. The child would not exist, she explained, unless I made the decision to go the donor egg route. In this way the baby was different from an adopted child, who had already been brought into the world. Furthermore, the laws of the United States stated that an egg donor had no rights to the baby I would carry. The donor was just providing the genetic material for me and my husband. The baby would develop in my womb. I would give birth, and the baby would be totally mine.

I told the counselor that I adored my two children even though I was glad to be divorced from their father. I said at this point it was like the movie *Peggy Sue Got Married*. In that film Kathleen Turner travels back in time from a high school reunion to her real high school past. Peggy now knows with 20/20 hindsight that her husband will turn out to be a bastard. However, she does not choose differently, because if she did, her two children would no longer exist. Similarly, I was glad to have chosen Pierre, even knowing my marriage would have a painful ending. Without Pierre I never would have had my two children, Elizabeth and Lisette.

With this line of thinking, I now had an epiphany. I realized that once I had my egg donor child and loved him or her, I would not want to go back, to somehow wish for a better technology that would have allowed me to use my own egg. Once I had a child, who cared about the egg source? At that moment I had a vision of a child that looked like my husband's baby picture. Currently Gabriel had very little hair. However, in the childhood photos on his mother's dresser, blond curls framed his face. That could be our child, I thought—curls all over and a resemblance to my husband. I wasn't a hundred percent about a donor egg, but I now felt that probably it could turn out well.

Lisette's bat mitzvah placed a timeline on everything. Now that I was proceeding with my donor, I was doing everything backward, processing my ambivalence after I already had committed to going the donor egg path.

Soon after my meeting with the psychologist, I was sitting alone at home. The children were at school, and I was enjoying a moment in the best room of our house, the step-down living room with cathedral ceilings. The bell rang twice. I opened the door, but no one was there. Instead I saw what looked like a giant crock-pot that came up to my knees. The FedEx tag had my husband's name on it. I called him at work to inquire about the delivery.

Apparently the new doctor wanted Gabriel's sperm checked by a place in the Midwest that conducted tests for sperm fragmentation. This outfit had delivered a huge container filled with liquid nitrogen to our front door. Gabriel, at his pleasure, would deposit his semen in a specially provided plastic test tube. Afterward the tube and its precious cargo would be preserved by the liquid nitrogen. Gabriel would just dial up FedEx and they would pick up his sample. In a few weeks, we would learn if Gabriel's sperm were fragmented. I hoped that they were normal, but it was nice for once to have the focus turned on his bodily products rather than on my rotten eggs.

Meantime Gabriel's parents were also patiently awaiting the arrival of their grandchild. They were given updates after each IVF trial. They knew that our chances were better this time because we were using a donor egg. Gabriel's father, Abe, was still feisty, still belting out "Hava Nagila" as he pushed his walker to the dialysis machine.

One day the nurses hooked him up, and two hours into the treatment the doctor stopped by. "How's it going, Abe?"

"It's going great, Doc. I'll be ninety-seven in a week. I feel fine."

"Well, you're looking good."

"Glad to hear it. Happy Purim, Doc!"

At that moment Abe keeled forward. His blood pressure plunged, and his pulse disappeared. The nurses and doctor struggled to insert a breathing tube to put Abe on a respirator. He was also in a coma.

Gabriel was called at work. He drove the hour and a half to the hospital. On the way, he picked up his mother, Eve. The live-in health aide, Wanda, wanted to come too. The doctor told them that unless Abe woke up soon, the prognosis was very poor.

Eve wheeled her walker to her husband's bedside. She took Abe's hand.

"Abe, wake up. It's Eve. I love you. Please wake up."

Wanda tried a different approach. "Abe, it's morning. I made your favorite oatmeal. Wake up now. Time to rise and shine."

Then Gabriel, Eve, and Wanda broke into a spirited rendition of "Hava Nagila." They sang their hearts out. But Abe did not awaken.

Within a few days, Abe was gone. He had left instructions to pull the plug once there was no hope. Now he himself could never have a chance to hold his grandchild. But if the donor egg baby was conceived, Abe's scholarly line would acquire its ninth-generation descendant. At Lisette's bat mitzvah we would dedicate "Hava Nagila" to Abe.

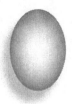

Should I Stay or Should I Go?

The egg donor agent called and said, "Don't freak out when you check your e-mail." My donor was having second thoughts, she explained. The good news was that she passed her physical exam the day before and was accepted as a patient by my new egg donor doctor. The bad news was that once she fully understood what the process entailed, she wasn't sure that she wanted to continue.

Now that I had finally acquiesced to an egg donor, I expected a smooth ride. Instead the ride had gotten even bumpier. Instead of my defective, aged egg, now I might not have any egg at all.

Luckily the agency smoothed everything over. They spoke to the donor and reassured her about the procedures. The California doctor's office also called her and explained what to expect in a tranquil manner. She agreed to continue.

My local hospital, the one where I had my last failed IVF attempt, was monitoring me as agreed. Unfortunately, one of their doctors—the debonair one—located a cyst on my right ovary. This doctor could not predict what would happen because I was officially the patient of the physician in California. Later I called the California office and was told by the assistant that I might not be able to proceed. Now I was afraid that, however fertile my twenty-something-year-old donor's eggs were, my forty-something-year-old womb would not be in shape to accept them.

Everything went back on track. Miraculously my cyst disappeared.

The recently started Lupron shot the growth into oblivion.

My new California IVF donor doctor advocated Spartan living—even before the embryos were transferred into me. No sex, drugs, or rock and roll. My husband and I were placed on a lovemaking moratorium. No alcohol or caffeine allowed either, and the doctor had to clear all exercise. Swimming, jumping on a trampoline, and ice-skating were out. No perfume, sprays, or powders, and I could not use cleaning products—at least my husband would have to be less demanding about how clean the house was! I was supposed to avoid stress (fat chance, considering the way my donor egg cycle had been progressing). Next I expected the doctor to tell me to become a vegan and to meditate three times a day. At this point I was desperate enough to try anything.

Gabriel was leaving in three days. The plane reservations were confirmed. He'd be going ahead to eject his sperm. Then he could sit by the pool for four days sunning and drinking piña coladas until I arrived.

I'd be home popping pills. I was taking antibiotics to prevent infection, steroids to keep androgen levels low, baby aspirin to maximize uterine blood flow, and prenatal vitamins to nurture the upcoming baby. Once Gabriel departed, I'd be a single mother again.

In the meantime, I packed my suitcase. I was bringing tank tops, capris, and skirts for the warmer weather. Gabriel booked an inn in the center of a quaint California town. That way he could carry me back good food from the romantic restaurants. I'd be imprisoned in the bed. The "stress-free living" donor doctor required me to sit in the bed for three days after the egg transfer: he was of the same school as Lauren, who spent a week in bed with her legs up after every IVF cycle. And again there would be no sex, drugs, or rock and roll. The aphrodisiac atmosphere of the hotel room would be wasted. I hoped I'd see a little of the town before the eggs were ready for their new home.

The girls would be abandoned. Once I left, I wouldn't be back for six days. There would be a three-day possible transfer period, and then three days allotted for bed rest. I found a babysitter to sleep over the first three days, and my parents would be back from Florida to watch for the last three. I also told Elizabeth and Lisette that if I could find them sleepover dates, they could stay with their friends during the weekend rather than having the babysitter. Elizabeth had her own thoughts.

"Mom, I don't need a babysitter. I'll stay home alone."

"I'm not leaving you home by yourself."

"Don't you trust me?"

"Of course I trust you. What if a robber breaks in the house at night?"

"There won't be a robber. You don't trust me!"

"Look, it's not a matter of not trusting you. Besides you'll be by yourself during the day, and I'm not worried about what you'll do."

Then I thought, oops—now I gave her the idea of having the entire day to herself. She'd invite the whole high school to a wild afternoon party. They'd trash the house, raid the wine rack, drag race down our road mowing down the neighbors' children. When Gabriel and I returned, the police would be waiting to arrest us for giving liquor to minors. I'd have to call frequently to Elizabeth's cell phone from my hotel bed to check for the background noise of reveling teenagers.

I did not tell my daughters that I was using an egg donor. I did not want to increase their negativity toward the baby. I was afraid that they would declare that since there was no blood relationship, the baby was not even their sibling. Also, I did not want them involved in my donor choice. When I took them shopping with me, they always made fun of every outfit I tried on. What if they rejected the donor I'd picked and demanded I select a different one? It was easier just to tell them that I was flying to California to be treated by a really good infertility doctor. That went over fine, and I don't think they suspected anything. If I eventually did become pregnant, I would "fess up."

The call from the out-of-state nurse interrupted my parental reverie.

"Your final ultrasound is superb. Your lining is just right. Keep all medication levels the same."

"I'm glad everything is going so well. Gabriel's getting ready to leave soon."

"We saw the donor today. We're doubling her medication. If that doesn't work we're canceling the cycle."

"What?"

"The donor isn't responding properly and her estrogen level is too low."

"Isn't there anything to take out?"

"There are a few follicles but they are immature. We'll know Monday if we can proceed. So have a nice weekend and don't worry about it yet."

Don't worry about it! How could there be no eggs? She was in her twenties. What did it matter how great my lining was if there was nothing to put in it!

At three in the morning I was lying awake in my own bed, imprisoned by insomnia. The Passover song "Had Gadya"—"One Little Goat"—kept going through my head. I'd had the Seder at our house this year at Gabriel's request. That way he could bring his mother by car service and she wouldn't be alone for the first night of Passover, now that Abe was gone. We also invited my brother, sister-in-law, and two nieces, as well as my brother's mother-in-law. She too was widowed. At the end of the Seder, we all held paper Haggadahs and sang the Goat Song. Each verse featured animals who suffered unfortunate casualties, followed by the refrain, "My father bought for two zuzim: one little goat, one little goat." Now at three a.m. I was creating my own rendition. It went like this:

Then came a womb,
That had a cyst,
That was too old,
That was waiting for an egg,
From a reluctant donor,
My husband bought for 2K plus,
No little eggs, no little eggs.

Gabriel's bags were packed, and he was ready to leave on a jet plane. The sperm was his precious cargo. He also was transporting a pharmacy in his carry on. My Lupron and estradiol vial were stuffed in the bag. The needles were in his suitcase. Otherwise they'd be confiscated.

I had to take a crash course in giving shots. Until I joined Gabriel, I would be administering the Lupron shots in my stomach each night. I recruited a nice nurse from my local IVF hospital to give me the intramuscular estradiol injections. In fact all the donor egg nurses were especially sweet. They probably thought of us egg donor recipients as so low in the fertility success scale that we deserved more empathy. Now every few days I found myself in an office dropping my drawers and bending forward for the nice nurse to thrust a needle in my butt.

The doctor called Gabriel on his cell right before he boarded the plane.

"Don't go! Get off the plane! She is not a confirmed yes. She is a maybe."

Apparently our donor was still a possibility. Her follicles had expanded, but they were half the desired size and her estrogen had shot up fivefold. Maybe in the end she might produce beautiful eggs, but they seemed to require twice the preparation time of anyone else's. There was also a chance her follicle development would abort and stop progressing at all. In two days she'd return for an ultrasound. Then Gabriel could start hanging out at airports all over again.

Two days later the phone rang at home.

"Victoria? Hello. I'll put the doctor through to you."

"Is she a go?"

"I don't know. One minute, please."

I ran downstairs to hand Gabriel the other phone. He was in his basement bachelor pad, waiting at home for the news, ready to hop in the car and dash to the airport for a stand-by flight.

"Victoria," the doctor said, "I just saw the donor."

"Is she a yes? Are there eggs?"

"No, the cycle is canceled."

"Oh God, no. But they were growing."

"They stopped progressing and haven't changed for two days."

"Can't you give her more medication and get them growing again?"

"No. If you retrieve eggs that stopped growing they are abnormal. They'll be blackened. The good news is that she had an exam two days ago and got a hundred on it."

"That's great."

Who cared if she got a hundred on her test! I knew that she was smart when I picked her! Now all of her intelligence wasn't going to benefit me. Her eggs would stay in her own body. My Cadillac Seville plush lining would remain empty.

Gabriel and I hugged each other. This was the first time we were actually together for one of the bad news phone calls. The sadness was as overwhelming as with my own five failed egg cycles. I had just lost my sixth baby.

Gabriel and I left to commiserate. I gave the children a quick pizza dinner beforehand. Then we escaped to the privacy of a booth at TGI Fridays, where we could talk without Elizabeth and Lisette eavesdropping.

I ordered a glass of wine, now that I was no longer under the orders of my teetotaling doctor. Gabriel, who rarely drinks, ordered the jumbo beer. The somber mood of our table did not match the beer guzzlers screaming at the bar. Our waitress probably thought we were getting a divorce or that someone had died.

We both were shocked. How could this have happened? Even my forty-plus-year-old eggs had always made it out and back in again. *They* never stalled and turned colors in my ovaries. For a wild moment we were tempted to escape the black hole of our missing baby. We considered using my not yet canceled plane tickets, buying Gabriel new ones, and vacationing at the inn that was still waiting for our arrival.

Then Gabriel thought about the finances. He started calculating all of our costs on a cocktail napkin. Shopping for eggs was strictly an "as is" proposition. Buyer beware: you paid something even if there was no baby, and you paid if there were no eggs. Sure, there would be a refund for the prepaid surgical procedures that were never performed, and for most of the donor's fee. Still, we were out almost ten thousand dollars for the evaluations, medications, and office visits of the donor with the midget eggs. Then there were the airfares and the nonrefundable hotel room. Not to mention the thousands more we had already gambled on my own five barren attempts.

Gabriel was wavering. Maybe we should halt the quest for a baby and terminate the bloodline of scholars. The prospect of us becoming paupers was eroding his sense of procreative duty.

I did not want to stop. Despite my donor egg ambivalence, I wanted to try the method at least once. If we failed, I wanted it to be because our last-ditch donor egg effort truly did not work, not because we never got the eggs.

Later that night, we finally broke the doctor's moratorium on lovemaking. I was hopeful my superlative uterine lining would create a miracle. Maybe we'd get pregnant on our own! Then I remembered that the Lupron had suppressed ovulation. My husband's sperm were playing Marco Polo with nonexistent eggs.

Chapter Eight

Breeding Babies

Back to the Mall—May 2005

abriel's baby lapse was temporary. A few days later he still wanted a child. I believed I still wanted an actual baby and not just the satisfaction of becoming pregnant. I avoided the pain of facing my donor egg loss by switching into action mode. Once again I was glued to my computer chair and surfing the web. The search was on for another donor. Now I had a new requirement. The prospective donor had to be experienced. I wanted someone who not only had previously donated Grade A, "unblackened" eggs, but whose eggs had gotten someone pregnant. This forced me to look only at the deluxe category of "extraordinary" or "premier" donors. My successful donor also had to be bright; the only premier characteristic I wasn't demanding was that she look like or actually be a model. Demanding two out of three desirable donor traits meant we were talking major bucks. Soon we would have to take out a loan or refinance our home.

The cheapest path was to use our previous agency. Their agency fee was going to be lost no matter what, but at least it could be applied toward a new donor. We found one donor who looked promising. Her eggs had impregnated women before. She was local and could be brought into my own IVF facility. She was bright and also had exceptional athletic and musical talent.

If she worked out, I decided I would have to expose my toddler to both sports and music. I would buy him, her, or them soccer balls. If they were adept at kicking the ball, I would join the preschool leagues and finally become an aggressive soccer mom. Then I would try piano and Suzuki violin lessons. Being tone deaf, I would find it difficult to determine if my children were talented. With Elizabeth and Lisette it had been easier, since both had quit every instrument they ever started in elementary school.

Alas, my athletic, musical diva egg donor was eliminated. She had donated five times previously and my local hospital did not allow more than four donations, since more than that might compromise the donor's ability to have her own children.

By now I was coming to think that we "mature" IVF patients deserved receiving a commission from the fertility doctors. First, we guaranteed them repeat business because the odds that we would succeed with our own eggs were staggeringly against us. Next, once we resorted to the donor egg option we spent even more money. Then, when the young donors who had provided us with all their multiple egg donations themselves suffered from infertility for having done so, they themselves became the physicians' next crop of IVF candidates.

I continued my donor search. Two other promising donors were ruled out: one because she "was retiring" after her sixth cycle; the other because having already donated four times, she now had a waitlist of twelve people. This last candidate was a very pretty student at an Ivy League college. Her evening gown photo displayed a bulging bust. The agency questionnaire required her to reveal whether the breasts were natural or silicon: hers were the real McCoy. True, her teeth were a bit crooked, but braces might fix that!

The hormones finally took their toll on my figure. My sixth treatment cycle, in preparation for my no-show egg delivery, had done me in. I now weighed more than I had ever weighed except when I was pregnant. When I went to a disco fundraiser at my children's school, I had to be creative with my costume. Although I still fit into my leather top with gold brocade from the eighties, the matching leather skirt was a lost cause. I compromised by finding a "back of the closet," loose-fitting skirt with faux fur. Gabriel discovered an outfit that he wore to the discos thirty years ago. He fit into his seersucker jacket and polyester pants with ease.

One offering at the "silent" auction fundraiser was a husband-and-wife membership at a local health club valued at eight hundred dollars.

I decided that since I was between IVF cycles and on a delay because of Lisette's bat mitzvah, I should focus on winning this item and fixing my figure. I bid fifty dollars and figured I'd obtained the best buy of the night. As soon as the loudspeaker announced that the auction would be closing, a woman stepped up to my bid sheet and entered the requisite ten-dollar increase. I pounced on the sheet and bid seventy. My competitor suggested we pool resources: we could purchase the membership together and join the health club as "a couple." I thought that was a great idea. We'd win via cooperation instead of competition. The next day we arrived at the health club office. We were honest and told them we were not gay but that we had excluded our husbands in order to join together.

My first day of working out at the health club I wore shorts and a T-shirt. When I arrived at the class, the women were well coiffed. Their hair was blow-dried, their nails painted, and they wore skimpy designer outfits. No one was overweight. In fact the women looked like they were competing for the title of "Miss Anorexia."

The class started well. I marched on the step and did jumping jacks. We needed to stay in place because the tiny room was filled to capacity with exercising women. Then the instructor began hollering out moves like a square dance caller. "Reverse turn," "Pivot turn," and "Around the world," she yelled. My fellow steppers gracefully performed the desired maneuvers. I turned the wrong way, bumped into the people on either side of me, and collided with the instructor in front. I was right behind the teacher, so all the other participants, not to mention the next class already lined up behind the glass partition and watching, had a great view of all my missteps. I was tempted to walk out, but there was no clear path. It felt like being at the junior high school mixer and not being able to dance. Finally the class ended. I resolved to try "spinning" on the exercise bicycle next time.

Besides making me gain weight, the IVF regimen was also causing me to lose my hair. Although my mother's hair had become very thin after delivering my brother and me, my own hair had remained thick after two deliveries. Now, however, with my body placed into ready mode for six additional pregnancies, I was beginning to see my scalp through my hair. If I finally became pregnant, I'd have nine more months of hair thinning. I was afraid that at the end I'd be totally bald. If so, for the next Hollywood theme fundraiser, Gabriel and I could both go as Yul Brenner from *The King and I*.

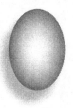

Egg Fight

When my California student donor didn't produce the eggs, the doctor from there recommended I use her again. He seemed certain that it was stress that had done in her eggs and that if she hadn't had her university exam that week, she would have been fine. I did not want to risk another ten-thousand-dollar failure and end up back at TGI Friday's providing the waitresses with another glum dinner scene. The agency we'd used continued to have faith in this donor, still listing her in their selection pool with no comment about her tiny eggs or previous failure. The California doctor also told me that five months before Lisette's bat mitzvah date should be a "safe" time to transfer and ensure that I still could make it to her event. That meant I had to wait six months.

The evening after my talk with the doctor, I went on my first donor egg chat room. The leader of the chat was a representative from a donor egg agency. Besides providing us with information, she could promote her agency. In order to join the chat, you had to enter a user name. Some people used a first name. Other chose an apropos alias such as "Donor Hunter" or "Good Egg." Then you typed in your questions and waited for the agent to respond.

One person complained that she couldn't locate any Jewish eggs. The agent referred her to two New York Orthodox agencies that sold only Jewish eggs. The catch: you probably had to be an Orthodox Jew to be qualified for such eggs.

Ever concerned with intelligence, I asked about verification of a donor's academic record. A reputable agency always documented such academic achievements, claimed the chat room leader.

Another seeker of Jewish eggs wanted to know how you could know if the donor was really Jewish. You could meet her, the agent recommended. And do what? I wondered. Ask them Torah questions? Even bona fide Jews might not know much "Torah trivia." In that case, the representative said, it was a "leap of faith." I had never thought of the possibility that the donor might lie about being Jewish. Hadn't Henry IV, the Protestant pretender to the throne of France, decided "Paris is worth a Mass" and become a Catholic to become king? Why couldn't Christian or Muslim donors become "online Jews" if by doing so they would command higher prices?

A few weeks later I attended another chat room discussion. This one was about gestational reduction, a program that "knocked off" some embryos when the fertility treatment resulted in too many. The leader of our group was supposed to "arrive" at eight p.m. By 8:15, there was no leader. The other participants began transmitting messages like:

"Where is the leader?"

"Do you think she is a no-show?"

By 8:30 we began our own leaderless chat. Soon we diverged from the reduction topic and began telling our own fertility stories. I exchanged e-mail addresses with one of the participants.

Later this woman told me via cyberspace that she too was looking for an egg donor. Her egg donor would have to sign a contract that she'd be available in the future to meet the child, since the woman thought it would be in the best interest of her child to know in person the identity of his or her egg mother.

I emphatically told her that I wanted just the opposite. I would see any donor who showed up at my doorstep as a stalker. Once the egg was donated, I wanted her to feel no further connection to it. My husband and I would be forever grateful, but the donor would not be a part of our lives.

I compared shopping tips with my e-mail donor egg colleague as we searched for eggs on the computer. She had been hunting for someone with dark brown hair, and I had been looking at the blondes.

Then one day my fellow shopper called.

"Victoria, I found someone!"

"That's great!"

"I just put down the deposit to hold her. I'm her last donation."

"I found someone too. At last the kids are going to visit their dad so Gabriel and I can discuss the donor this weekend."

"My donor is pretty and smart."

"So is mine," I echoed.

"I used the agency you told me about."

"I'm using them too."

"I had to compromise. The donor isn't brunette."

"That's funny. Mine isn't blonde either."

"What page is your donor on? I'll look her up."

"She's on page three," I replied.

"So is mine. Which one is she?"

"The one with the red hair," I elaborated.

"That's the donor I just booked!"

"You're kidding!"

"No, I'm serious," she said.

"Did you definitely book her?'

"Yes."

"If you change your mind let me know."

Now I had lost my donor eggs again! I'd been sniped! Next time I wouldn't share so much information.

That Saturday Gabriel and I sat in bed sipping wine. We were buried in shopping bags full of photos and profiles of prospective donors. The children had finally left to be with their father for Memorial Day weekend, so Gabriel and I could do some serious searching.

I showed him all of the donor candidates. Gabriel didn't mind that we had lost the redhead because no one in our families had red hair. After much looking, we found one who was very promising. Then Gabriel asked the question dear to his heart: How much did she cost?

Gabriel almost fell out of the bed when he heard her fee was almost twenty thousand dollars. I pointed out to him that he needed to become an educated consumer. Hospitals had recently raised payments to the donors from seven to eight thousand dollars. Most agencies paid more than a hospital. Donors who had a proven record of impregnating women and were attractive and smart often charged fifteen thousand or more. Some of the more popular donors with a huge waitlist charged upward of twenty-five thousand. On top of the donor's fee, the agency charged either half of the donor's cost or a flat rate.

Gabriel drew a spending line. "There is only a fifty/fifty chance this is going to work anyway. I'm not paying over twenty thousand for the donor and the agency plus ten thousand for the medical costs. Even then we might end up with nothing but an even bigger debt."

"Then how do you suggest we do it?"

"Something will have to go."

We went back to the paper piles to study cost reduction. One possibility was to pick an "undesirable" trait. We could pick someone who might replace the Duchess of York as the next Weight Watchers' spokesperson. Or we also could pick someone who had suboptimal SAT scores and less than a 2.0 college GPA. There were always the faces that rivaled that of my great-grandmother Rivka. Rivka's girth *and* her countenance would save us a lot of money.

Gabriel didn't want to compromise on any desirable personal trait, but he also didn't want to break the bank. The only solution, in that case, was to revert to our previous approach: to find a person with "in demand" attributes who had never donated before. A "virgin" donor was much cheaper. I was reluctant to travel this route. We might have another bright student with a perfect score on her exam and eggs that went MIA.

I would continue to search. Perhaps we would be very lucky and find a Filene's Basement price for a designer donor—maybe someone who was donating more out of the goodness of her heart than the need to fill her pocketbook.

With our new fiscal constraints, I needed to refine my shopping strategy. I decided it was time to apply prom dress shopping skills to my egg hunt. When I was in high school, many girls placed prom dresses on hold in two or three shops. They purchased four gowns but left the tags on so that three or, if necessary, four could be returned. Then everyone tried on their dresses and polled their friends for the ultimate winner. I decided I could employ the same approach. I would put a number of donors on hold.

On the web pages of potential donors of one agency, I at first found no one appropriate for me, until I looked more closely. There she was—the very last one. She looked like me. Her hair, skin, and eye color matched mine, and the shape of her eyes was identical to mine.

My former criterion was to match my children. What if I focused on my own looks instead? When I went to the Chinese restaurant with my daughters, the waitress always asked, "Are those really yours?" My own parents told me unabashedly that the girls looked absolutely nothing like me. Now, with a donor egg, I might finally have a child who looked just like me.

This donor was also smart. Currently, though, she was "in cycle." She probably cost a fortune. I called the agency. "I like your last listed donor. How much does she cost?"

"She's comparable with the clinic rates."

"That's wonderful. But why?"

"She has relatives who were conceived by donor eggs and wants to help others do the same."

"Wow. That's really nice of her. Is she available after her cycle?"

"Let me see if there's a waitlist. You can be first on the list. But you may not be able to get her."

"Why not?"

"We don't want our donors to feel like part of a factory. So I won't ask her if she wants to donate again until two weeks after her current cycle ends."

I was impressed that this agency actually treated their donor as something other than a money breeder. I told the agent that I would wait for this donor. But I would not count on her. For one thing she would have to agree to donate again. And if her current donation failed to create a pregnancy, we wouldn't use her.

Meanwhile, I continued to look for other donors to add to my shopping cart. From a different agency I located another donor with my hair color and my college major. When the extra photos arrived via e-mail, I recognized her as someone I'd seen before online with another agency. Indeed, some donors could be found in five or more agencies. The price might vary from agency to agency, as could the agency cost. Comparison shopping, even for the same donor, could save a lot of money.

The donor photos that were sent via e-mail weren't flattering. However, the picture on the donor's new agency was very pretty. It was probably professionally done. I was enthralled and wanted to reserve this donor too. With her prior agency and photos she had never been chosen, but now she was suddenly in demand. For five hundred dollars, I too could hold a place on her waitlist. I was ready to proceed. Gabriel, however, said no. Despite the donor's new, spiffy look, he could not forget her original photos. He noticed the moles that had been covered with make-up on her more recent, touched-up headshot. Gabriel was becoming pickier and pickier. I would have to shop further.

Finally I found another donor from a different agency. This one looked like my children. She lived in the middle of the plains, and there were no IVF egg centers near her. We would definitely have to fly her to egg donor civilization. Like my other possible donor, she was in the midst of growing eggs for another recipient. If her crop was successful, she too would be a possibility. Now I had two "prom queens" on hold who could become the egg mother of my child. If neither worked I would have to locate a third possibility. If they both came through, I'd probably choose the most recent find because I still preferred the donor to resemble my children. Plus this donor had a big selling point. She had spent time in Disneyland playing Cinderella. I figured if she was good enough for Walt Disney standards, then she was good enough for me!

Gabriel was still holding up well considering all those failed trials and the death of his father. He was happy that our next trial would again be with a donor egg. Even under stress, Gabriel was very predictable. He ate one kind of cereal each morning. At lunch he mashed tuna from a can, added mayonnaise, and plopped it on two pieces of toast. His sock and underwear drawers were each neatly arranged by color. When he placed Snapple jars in the recycle bin, he meticulously lined them up in rows.

Gabriel was also financially conservative. He had saved for years so that he could buy a house if he ever found a wife. When I came along with the children, we pooled resources. The house was the smallest on the block, but in a good school district. The main drawback, as we subsequently learned, was that because the backyard was the size of a plastic kiddy pool, we could not meet the building code if we tried to build an extra bedroom for a third child.

Instead of concentrating on how we might expand our existing real estate, Gabriel came to me with the "breaking news" that he was ready to purchase a place in Paris! Gabriel had read in the *New York Times* that Americans were flocking to Paris to buy apartments. They purchased them in their fifties, held onto them as an investment, and retired there in their sixties. While I researched possible egg donors on the internet, Gabriel gazed nightly at Parisian apartments. We could refinance our home to afford the downpayment on the apartment. After we bought it, we could rent it out for additional income.

Gabriel was ready to buy a cheap plane ticket for an overnight package deal in Paris. We could fly most of the night, arrive in France at dawn, shop for apartments the remainder of the day, and fly home the next afternoon. It seemed to me that Gabriel, like the stereotypical Catholic kid who goes to a strict parochial school and then goes wild in college, had "lost it." At least his midlife crisis seemed to involve an apartment rather than a mistress.

I, the impractical dreamer of babies produced with forty-plus-year-old eggs, became the voice of reason.

"Gabriel, we can't buy a French apartment now. I may get pregnant with donor eggs. We might have twins! We don't have enough bedrooms for one baby, let alone two."

In fact Gabriel was probably preparing his "Plan B." His neat plan for the universe had included first obtaining the wife, then producing a baby. That was still a question mark, and if the question mark became a definitive "no," Gabriel would need something to keep from falling apart. The Parisian apartment was the cushion to ease his fall. We hoped the donor egg would work, and Gabriel's equanimity wouldn't be tested. It was unlikely that the next donation would proceed as badly as the last one.

In the meantime I was still researching fertility findings. One day in the *New York Times*, I read that bone marrow had been reported to contain stem cells that produced brand new eggs for the ovaries, possibly even in women undergoing menopause.

Of course, almost the entire scientific world of fertility specialists had disputed these findings, adhering to the party line that all women were born with all of their eggs, which gradually "rotted" as one got older. One lone dissenter from a prestigious institution felt that the discovery had merit.

In the past I would have been on the phone calling the bone marrow researchers, even offering myself as a guinea pig in the first stem cell baby making trial. The fact that I did not pursue the procedure further was a litmus test that proved how far I had come toward accepting a donor egg. I felt more at peace, especially now with my Cinderella donor. I already had developed affection for her eggs and the future offspring they might generate. The need to use my own egg did not seem as pressing.

I still had a nagging doubt. What if I was to become part of a narrow sliver of time, part of a group of women who had borne the soon-to-be-extinct species of donor egg babies. We would be the dinosaur products of a short blip of insufficient technology. After us, every infertile mother had benefited from the bone marrow technique, and a whole generation of eighty-year-old mothers were now wheeling themselves in wheelchairs beside the strollers in which sat their brand-new-egg babies.

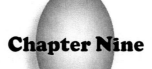

Chapter Nine

Is That Your Final Egg?

Upper East Side in New Jersey—July 2005

The agency from my Cinderella candidate had been very conscientious. They e-mailed or called me every few days with an egg update from her current donation. Apparently the recipient couple already had performed two home pregnancy tests before the scheduled blood test and both tests were positive! This donor might eliminate my usual agony of waiting with nihilistic desperation for the white background to turn pink.

The next day I learned the official blood pregnancy test results for my number one donor choice. She had made her egg recipient pregnant!

Now that we had found our donor, we once again had to choose a transfer site. This time we wouldn't be flying to the donor, since she already had to ride far across the plains to a satellite egg-monitoring station. Gabriel finally found an acceptable facility in New Jersey that would cut our costs because they required a shorter donor stay. The donor's preference was to come during the two weeks of her college vacation, right after the Christmas holidays. I would try to accommodate her. My potential motherhood would be delayed again. However, I would then look less pregnant at Lisette's bat mitzvah.

Finally, after a month of waiting, I had my first appointment at the new IVF location. Gabriel was able to take off time, and we went together. The lobby featured an Au Bon Pain restaurant with its round black metal tables and individual yellow umbrellas. The waiting room had a large aquarium so I could be soothed by the fish while I waited for the doctor. There also was a machine that spouted free coffee, tea, and hot chocolate. When they called my name, they used the more anonymous "Victoria H" so that not every waiting room inhabitant would be able to identify me. This was five-star baby making in New Jersey!

The doctor had actually read my chart, which was now a tome, beforehand. He complimented me on having tried five times on my own. He said that showed real commitment and that I had thoroughly pursued the biological route before switching to the egg donor path.

Just in case there was hope after all for my own egg, I couldn't resist asking him about the latest stem cell research. "Am I just missing the boat by not waiting for the bone marrow stem cell research to be completed?"

"No. First of all, this is the wrong White House administration for stem cell research. Even the states like California that are passing local laws for stem cell research don't have the federal funding they'll need to conduct the research. And it could still take another five or six years to complete the studies."

"I just thought I'd ask." I sighed.

"Egg donation is your only real option now. If the donor egg goes to the five-day blastocyst stage your chances of pregnancy will be 70 percent. Even if we transfer at day three we still have a 60 to 65 percent success rate at our facility."

After the doctor meeting, we went to see the psychologist, who was a tall, comely woman. She wanted to know if we'd tell the child that he or she was conceived by another's egg. I said that I didn't want any family secrets and that I would tell the child as well as Elizabeth and Lisette. The psychologist then showed us her collection of egg donor books that explained to the child that it came from its father's sperm and another mother's egg.

The psychologist also provided pointers about locating an egg donor. She said it was important to look not just at the donor's photo but at photos of her whole family. After all, the donor might be a beautiful, blonde Marilyn planted in the middle of the Munster family. She then invited us to join a four-session group for couples planning to utilize donor eggs. Gabriel and I agreed to attend.

She waved goodbye when we left, and the nurses also waved goodbye as we passed through the door. I felt as if we were in Oz being pampered to meet the wizard.

The question that nagged me the most now was my age. Fifty seemed too old for embarking on motherhood again, and I was rapidly approaching that milestone. I would be impregnated with the baby right before my forty-eighth birthday and delivering when I was almost forty-nine. By the time the child graduated from high school, I would be close to seventy. Since my hormones had been good and my flow had not dried up, I didn't feel that this pregnancy was going against my body. I knew that the technology allowed menopausal women in their sixties to conceive, but I didn't want to be one of them. I had my own internal biological clock. Fifty was the point at which I knew I would feel like a freak of nature if I somehow defied the fertility gods and became pregnant.

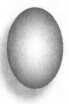

Life and Death

N ow that the baby might finally become a reality, it seemed time to check in again with our current family. Once the children returned from camp, Gabriel made a real effort to spend more time with them. He began by buying tickets for a Mets game. The last time I had gone to a baseball game my brother was an aspiring player and Tom Seaver was pitching for the Mets. Elizabeth and Lisette, in contrast, had been to no ball games.

When we arrived at the game, it was "bobblehead" night. Lisette was given a free ceramic figure of a well-known pitcher with the head suspended on a spring that bobbed up and down. It was like the boy-and-girl "kissing" dolls that people used to display in their rear car windows. Elizabeth was mad that she didn't get one too, but she no longer looked twelve or under. (Elizabeth did not actually want the doll—she just wanted to leave it in its original box for extra value and then sell it on eBay for pocket money.)

In the time since I was a kid, the producers of baseball games had learned to keep the attention of everyone—even my blasé girls—with outsized electronic video games. Elizabeth and Lisette watched unsuspecting audience members caught on the overhead screen, they played games on the overhead screen such as figuring out which of the three moving hats ended up covering the baseball, and they scrambled for a souvenir during the T-shirt launch.

All went well until the Mets hit their sixth run, which was a homer. At that point a giant plastic apple emerged from a plastic hat on the ground and the streaking colors of fireworks streamed across the sky, followed by loud booms! At that, Elizabeth ran screaming out of the stadium. I found her hiding with her hands covering her ears by the indoor popcorn stand. She was terrified of fireworks. I finally convinced her to return by telling her that since the game was almost over, neither team was likely to make any more home runs. I was right, but since the Mets won, at the end of the game there was another crescendo of fireworks. Once more Elizabeth ran hollering out of her seat. Still, overall, the game was a hit.

Gabriel's next family project was a game of Monopoly minus Elizabeth, who did not want to play. Lisette was delighted. What with Gabriel's work schedule (which still hadn't improved) and the general lengthy play time of Monopoly, the board remained on the living room floor for three weeks as the game slowly progressed.

The latest kink to work out was how to address Gabriel. Lisette still called him Dad. Elizabeth alternated between Dad and Gabriel. In an effort to avoid the choice, she had taken to calling him "Hey you." Gabriel wanted me to intervene. He didn't care if Elizabeth called him Gabriel, but he wanted a name. I relayed the message to Elizabeth and gave her permission to call him Gabriel with the knowledge that she wasn't hurting his feelings.

In sum, I thought we were doing pretty well. Except that soon I would have to tell them I was trying for a baby again. That news never went over well. I'd also have to decide at what point to tell them that this time it was not my own egg.

Gabriel's mother was still waiting for a grandchild. Unlike Elizabeth and Lisette, she was eager for the baby's arrival. She was a strong woman and had beat five cancers, starting at age seventy-two. First, there had been cancer of the kidney, then blood cancer, breast cancer, lung cancer, and urethral cancer! Eve lost one kidney, one breast, and part of a lung from these malignancies. Her physical and emotional survival was nothing short of miraculous. She remained calm under the siege of each tumor.

Her upbringing had not prepared Eve for adversity. She grew up rich and pampered by servants, as part of a larger family that owned five small-town department stores. One was in upstate New York, one was in the Midwest, two were in the South, and the remaining one was near the Jersey shore. Her parents, like her aunts and uncles, were the token Jews of the community. Eventually Eve left her small town behind and attended one of the Seven Sister schools.

Abe and Eve met about twenty years post-college at a lecture in New York City. Abe asked Eve to "cut out" and go for a drink. Abe drank beer and teetotaling Eve drank milk. They married not long afterward. Abe thought that he was marrying into money. However, all five family stores gradually went under in the fifties, and Abe became a jack of all trades. He was a lawyer, psychologist, builder, and soldier.

He retired in his sixties, just in time for Eve and Abe to follow Gabriel to college in Charleston. They bought an apartment near the campus. While Gabriel was at school, Eve conducted house tours at the local antebellum mansions and Abe read magazines. On weekends they spent time with Gabriel. Gabriel was more accepting than I would have been. If my parents had come to college with me, I would have disowned them.

Now Eve had just been diagnosed with her second lung cancer. At age ninety-two, surgery and chemotherapy were no longer options. This would be the one cancer that Eve would not be able to conquer. Perhaps she would last long enough to either greet a newborn grandchild or at least know I was carrying her descendant. I was not sure how well Gabriel would hold up once he lost his mother too. Of course a new baby would help him cope with the loss of his parents.

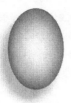

Door Number Two

For the first time I had an egg nightmare. In this dream, set in a cafeteria, I was the one donating the eggs. The recipient brought an entourage of rowdy friends and relatives to her egg transfer. We all followed the doctor to the cafeteria. The doctor positioned the recipient and me lengthwise on adjacent wooden cafeteria tables. We both had to sit up when our preparatory meal arrived—a thick, sweet potato soup. I don't like sweet potatoes and was terrified when the doctor demanded that we finish our soups.

Then I panicked and I realized that I'd forgotten to take my nightly anti-infection medication regularly. I admitted my lapse to the doctor.

"Doctor, I forgot to take the meds. But I have been taking allergy medication each day—Allegra or Benadryl. Does that count?"

"The Allegra won't fight an infection. The Benadryl might."

I asked the doctor hopefully, "You won't be operating on us right on the tables?"

"I've done plenty of operations on tables."

Next I started talking with the woman who was going to receive my egg.

"Right after I give you my eggs, I'm going to have someone else give me her eggs."

"That's amazing!" giggled the recipient.

The doctor ordered us to sit side by side on reclining cafeteria chairs. The only thing missing was the *Bride of Frankenstein* wires hooking my ovaries with hers.

The doctor said, "Now I'll have to check your vaginal fluid to make sure that there's no infection, since you didn't take your pills properly."

All of the recipient's nearest and dearest were looking on, waiting for me to undress and to have my fluid checked. My anxiety mounted as the nightmare set in: What if this was not a real doctor? What if these people were actually members of a satanic egg cult who were going to rip out my eggs, Manson–style.

A trickle of laughter penetrated the cafeteria. The giggling, whispering voice sounded like Elizabeth.

Then I clearly heard Elizabeth say, "You were really sleepwalking?"

Another female voice answered, "I do that sometimes."

Now I realized that Elizabeth and her girlfriend who was sleeping over were in my bathroom. Normally I would have been angry they were in there and had woken me up. This time I was grateful to be saved from the nightmare.

Gabriel missed the excitement of my nightmare because he had left early in the morning for shul. Every morning, for one year, he would say the Kaddish for his father. Lisette crawled into bed next to me soon afterward.

"Lisette, I had a bad dream. They were taking my eggs out in a cafeteria" (I left out the mutual donation part).

"I had a baby dream too a few nights ago."

"Really, what was it?" I asked.

"You, Dad, Elizabeth, and I were all on a plane going on a trip. We had a baby with us too. Then we couldn't find the baby. We all had to get off the plane and look for it."

"Did we find it?"

"No, it disappeared."

"That sounds like what you would really want to happen if there was a baby—vanish."

"Very funny."

When awake, and not having egg dreams, I was still vigilant for cutting-edge infertility discoveries. Later that day I read about stem cell findings in mice that one day might affect the health of any IVF baby. The stem cell line would come from each IVF baby. Fertilization outside the womb should allow for a cell to be taken off when the embryo reached eight cell divisions. This individual eighth cell could be developed into an entire embryonic stem cell line, and the other seven cells could still be implanted in the uterus and become a baby. The Right to Life movement should not object because the one cell technique left the embryo healthy and viable. If the baby grew up and suffered serious injuries, its stem cell line could always come to the rescue, providing new nerve endings and perhaps entire new bodies—a person could travel with his or her portable freezer filled with embryonic stem cells. The ever elusive fountain of youth really was becoming a Brave New World.

That same day *New York* magazine had an article about single women in their thirties freezing their eggs so that they'd have a better chance of pregnancy in the future. That way they could wait until their forties or fifties, obtain the pinnacle of their profession, or locate Mr. Right, before having babies. Of course even in their thirties they might not have good eggs, and the freeze-and-thaw technique might not be perfected enough for their eggs to work later. Apparently it was easier to freeze a fertilized egg that made it to the blastocyst stage rather than an unfertilized egg.

One morning the phone rang. Now that my pregnancy attempts had gone on hold, I no longer jumped every time I heard the phone ring. This call was from the hospital where I was on the waitlist.

The voice at the other end said, "We have your donor."

"What?"

"I know it's been a long time on the waitlist but we finally found you someone."

"Who?"

"A twenty-year-old woman who looks just like you."

"Really?"

"Yes, she could be your sister."

"In what way do we look alike?" I asked.

"You have an identical chin."

"Oh, I see," I responded.

"This donor loves to paint and draw and is quite artistic."

"Well that's nice. Did she also do okay in school?"

"I don't know. The hospital doesn't ask about academics. Sometimes the psychologist might mention if she thinks the person is bright or did well, but this report doesn't mention anything about her academic ability."

"Oh."

"Would you like to see her information? You have forty-eight hours to decide once you receive the packet. I can fax it or next-day deliver it. If you decline, you go back on the waitlist for the next available donor for you."

"I guess I'll accept the information. You might as well fax it now so I'm not in suspense."

"If you decide early that you don't want her, let me know because then we have to find a new match for her eggs. This is a shared cycle, so two of you will be using her."

Finally, after a year and a half, my hospital donor match was made. I waited eagerly by the fax machine. At this point I expected to proceed with my Cinderella donor, but I still wanted to see who my hospital match would have been. The fax machine began spewing fifteen pages. I read each one as it emerged.

The first pages were a description of the donor's appearance. Since there was no photo, each body part was described in multiple-choice detail by the donor—whether, for example, her nostril flare was "small, average, or wide." I was unable to envision how all the body pieces would fit together. Perhaps if I hired an artist who specialized in recreating criminal physiognomy from witness descriptions, I would have a picture of my donor. Meanwhile, this woman's chin, which was allegedly "identical" to mine, was described as having a "medium" cleft, a "square" shape, and a "strong" prominence. My chin had no cleft, little prominence, and was not square.

I was surprised that the donor was Ashkenazi Jewish on both sides. I had not listed religion as a criterion, so it seemed strange that they had matched me with her, especially since Jewish donors were in high demand. I liked her artistic abilities, but I wasn't sure if these could be inherited. Gabriel's mother had an apartment full of watercolors and oil paintings that she had copied from museum exhibits, but Gabriel would have trouble mastering a paint-by-number set. I missed the SAT scores and adult photos that agencies provided.

When Gabriel returned from work early that afternoon, I told him about the waitlist donor. We looked at the donor's and her family's physical appearance and medical history section, the list of her special skills, such as "manual dexterity," and the donor's psychological and genetic reports. Five year earlier, on Independence Day, the donor also reported she had smoked pot. Gabriel and I felt her honesty was commendable, but the admission did not bode well for her intelligence level.

Gabriel's strong inclination was to proceed with the agency donor. We had received and approved the contract drawn up by our lawyer, which she and her assigned lawyer (whose fees we also paid) were reviewing. Nothing had been signed yet, but we expected everything to move forward as planned.

Gabriel was home from work early because we were departing shortly for our first group session at the ritzy New Jersey clinic. As we were leaving, a nurse called to inform us that our Cinderella donor would need to fly out for her one-day evaluation before we could proceed. The nurse also explained the medication and egg stimulation schedule.

Then I called the agency and explained the projected schedule. The agent said the donor had an exact three-week time span in January; although the dates had to match precisely, she calculated that in fact we'd be off by two days. Still, we ought not to worry yet—the agent would call back and see if she couldn't work something out.

Not worry! I felt beaten down again. This felt too much like my "virgin" donor who first had not wanted to go through with it and then was unable to perform under stress. Now again my donor had a difficulty, in the form of a narrow time limit. What if her eggs weren't ready in time?

I was worrying the whole way on our drive to New Jersey for our donor egg group session. "Gabriel, maybe we should take the hospital's artistic donor. At least she's not on a three-week time line."

"Victoria, I'm sure the agency will work it out."

"I can't believe our second donor might fall off the donation map too."

"We don't know that yet."

"I'm sick of all these problems. Can't it just go smoothly for once?"

My cell phone rang. It was the agent. She was going to search for a facility that was willing to monitor me in Florida and was open during the holidays. That way I could spend my Christmas vacation getting my hormone shots and tests and be ready for the embryo transfer in New Jersey—assuming we stayed on the donor's timetable.

We soon arrived at our destination. The group consisted of the tall psychologist we had already met and five other couples. Everyone grabbed free drinks from the coffee machine and followed the psychologist into the conference room.

I was excited about this New Jersey group and the prospect of sharing our thoughts with other couples. I had some prior experience as a point of comparison. The other group meeting I had attended with Gabriel had featured an Australian speaker who had been impregnated with a donor egg in New York and given birth to twins. She felt privileged to have them, since Australia had outlawed paying for an egg (donors had to be willing to donate gratis), the government had to approve donor egg ads placed by prospective couples, and there was a seven-year wait for an egg. She and other Australians were flocking to American hospitals, which had no uniform regulations for the donor egg market.

My other group experience had been one for women who already had children and were proceeding with the donor egg option to obtain an enlarged family. We all had secondary infertility. This group didn't allow men to participate, and it ended prematurely because everyone in it, except me, became pregnant.

We all introduced ourselves and stated where we were in the infertility process. Gabriel and I were the furthest along—the only ones who'd actually tried a donor egg cycle, and the only ones who had definitely committed to using a donor egg. The other couples were only exploring the donor egg option. One couple had had their own egg and sperm transferred that morning at another facility, and they were hoping they wouldn't require the donor egg route. They told us that during their embryo transfer, their doctor had worn a black top hat, and that when the transfer was completed, he waved a magic wand over her abdomen. The group started laughing. The psychologist said she was pretty sure that she knew who their doctor was. The physician's outfit struck me as appropriately symbolic of the hocus pocus involved in the whole fertility process. I was glad, though, that so far none of my doctors had worn anything but a lab coat.

All of the other couples had no children. The psychologist led a discussion about how it felt to attend baby showers and to confront the holidays childless. I felt somewhat excluded from the conversation, since I was a mother already.

I shared an absurd example with the group. I told them that my children did not want a baby, only a puppy. We got the dog, and even though it wasn't my genes I still loved it. I was sure that if I could love a dog, I could love an infant even more. Someone in the group said it must be hard not to have my daughters' encouragement for having a new baby. I responded that I was used to it by now. I also felt accepted by the other members, even though I'd disclosed that I already had children.

At the end of the group, one of the couples started talking with Gabriel and me. The woman, a professor with a pageboy haircut and wire frame glasses, had hormone levels so abysmal that she couldn't even try with her own eggs.

She said, "I don't know if I feel comfortable using someone else's egg."

Her husband said, "I've told her you'll still be the mother."

"I'm not sure about a donor egg," replied the wife.

"I've tried to explain to her what makes a mother, and she'll still have everything that makes a mother," said the exasperated husband.

Gabriel, who was quiet during the group, pitched in now. "I think having the baby will be very rewarding in the end."

I thought that it was easy for the husbands to be so cavalier. It was still their genes. The donor egg scenario was very different from adoption, where both parties contributed no genetic material.

I told the couple that I had been informed that my age was too advanced.

The woman responded, "I know someone who had twins at age fifty."

"They must have used donor eggs," I said.

"The odds are overwhelming that it couldn't be her eggs at that age," added Gabriel.

"The fact that she had twins also suggests younger donor eggs," I said.

"I never thought of that," said the husband.

"All of the celebrities that are having babies at very late ages are using donor eggs—it just isn't advertised," I said.

Chapter Ten

To Be or Not To Be

Sperm Surprise–October 2005

The New Jersey nurse had made a recommendation. She said it was always a good idea to freeze some sperm as a backup. That way, if on the day of the egg retrieval Gabriel was unable to produce or "shot blanks," there would be alternative sperm.

Gabriel made an appointment for the upcoming weekend. He was able to schedule a Sunday afternoon and not have to miss work again. Then, after his specimen was delivered, he could visit his mother in New Jersey. She had survived the radio wave ablation of her tumor, and in a few months we would learn if it truly was destroyed.

When Gabriel returned Sunday evening, I asked him about his clinic appointment.

"Was it successful?"

"Yes."

"Did they only have one video in this place?"

"No, they had four."

"You must have been late getting to your mother's."

"I didn't watch the whole video, only selections."

"Were these selections oral sex again?"

"They were a mixture of everything."

"It sounds like you had an entertaining Sunday afternoon."

Five days later, when Gabriel returned from work, he told me that he had bad news for me.

"Victoria, they called about the sample I gave. There was a problem."

"What do you mean?"

"There were no sperm."

"What?"

"They couldn't find any sperm to freeze."

"What do you mean they couldn't find any? Did they lose them?"

"No. They said it was very easy to do a sperm count. It was zero."

"How could you not have any sperm?"

"I don't know."

"You've always had sperm. You had sperm all five times we used my eggs, and some of them always fertilized. You even had sperm for that stupid crock-pot that arrived at our door."

"There was a normal amount of fluid. There just wasn't any sperm in it. Maybe I didn't wait enough days from since we last had sex."

"What are we going to do?"

"They suggested that I see a male infertility specialist from our original hospital. I already scheduled a meeting with him. The soonest appointment is in two weeks. Meanwhile next week I'll give them another sample."

"Oh, God. Gabriel, I hope this is all a mistake."

"It's probably something the new place did differently, and that's why there were no sperm."

"Maybe the lab technician got distracted by one of the four porn videos and accidentally spilled your sperm."

I knew that Gabriel must have been devastated. All this time the focus had been on me and my overripe eggs. Finally, when the baby was in reach, Gabriel had zero sperm. If there were no sperm, he certainly could not continue his genetic line—or even try. What a blow to his manhood.

That night I couldn't sleep. I kept having a vision of a disheveled man sitting behind a table on a New York City street corner. He had arranged three white paper cups in a line across the table. Under one cup was an egg, under another cup a sperm, and under the third nothing. With great dexterity, the man continually changed the position of all three cups. My job was to watch carefully so that when the movement ended I could identify the sperm and egg cups. If I made the correct choice, I'd make a baby. But there also were trap doors with wind tunnels under the table. If the trap door opened under a cup and activated the wind tunnel, the sperm or egg would be blown away.

One week later Gabriel gave his sample and later that afternoon we drove to our next New Jersey group session.

"Both of these car rides to New Jersey have been terrible. On the way to the last group we didn't know if the scheduling dates of the donor would work for us. This time we don't know if we'll have any sperm," I complained.

"We'll know more in a day or two. I'll call to see if they found anything."

"Maybe we should talk about our options even if we don't know the answer to the sperm problem yet."

"Okay."

"One possibility is that we do it anyway and hope they find something the day of the egg retrieval."

"They also have a procedure where they can take sperm right out of the testes. They do a sperm biopsy. It only works, though, if they find sperm there," explained Gabriel.

"Maybe we could do that. But then we have the problem of where can we do that operation. The infertility doctor is at our first place, and they won't let us take in our own donor."

"Maybe they do sperm extraction in our new place too," said Gabriel.

"We could always adopt, but I know you said you wouldn't want to do that."

"I was thinking about it today. Maybe I would adopt."

"Another idea is to use sperm from one of your relatives."

"Yeah, I could use the sperm from one of my father's relatives."

"Why? So it would be related to your famous Jewish ancestor?"

"Yes. One of my relatives is a judge. He's a very prominent man."

"Was he at our wedding or Elizabeth's bat mitzvah?"

"He was at our wedding. We have a picture of him. He's a good-looking guy."

"You could ask him."

"Except he's almost sixty."

"I don't think they'll accept sixty-year-old sperm. Does he have any children?"

"He has one son who didn't come to our wedding. But the other son did. He also has a third child in California, but I think it's a girl."

"It would be weird at family gatherings. They'd all be looking at our child as their own child or grandchild."

"Yeah, it would be strange."

"We could also use a sperm bank. We could try to get something from you the day of the transfer, and if there was nothing we could use the backup donor sperm."

Gabriel's hands tightened on the steering wheel. His voice became louder and his eyebrows lowered.

"Victoria, you're being selfish. What's the matter with you? It took you five cycles to agree to a donor egg and now you're talking to me about some stranger's sperm."

"You brought up adoption. If you can adopt, then you can use someone's sperm. How dare you call me selfish! I'm the one who went through five IVF attempts for this baby, and now I've said I'll use someone else's egg."

"I don't want to talk about it any more."

"Okay, we won't."

"Maybe my count was zero because it was just low. Perhaps they measured a small sperm amount as zero."

"I thought you didn't want to talk about it anymore. You're in denial that you might have a problem. You're not ready to talk about it yet."

I was furious that Gabriel had called me selfish. I knew that he wasn't ready to deal with the possibility of having no sperm and no genetic child. Initially I had felt relieved about the possibility that he might consider adoption or donor sperm. We'd be on the "even playing field" the psychologist had talked about last week. We'd both be giving up our genetics to have a baby together. Then I felt guilty for that thought. Gabriel really wanted to have his own biological child. In fact, so did I.

After our group meeting, I asked the psychologist if we could meet alone with her for a few minutes. She agreed.

"We had a real shock," I said.

"When I went to freeze sperm, there weren't any. I just had a repeat test at a different facility this morning," elaborated Gabriel.

"I'm so sorry," said the psychologist.

"Do you know if someone here does the operation to retrieve sperm directly with a biopsy?" I asked.

"I'm not sure if we do."

"Also, do you ever have people who try to use their own sperm, but if it doesn't work they have a backup from a sperm bank?" I asked.

"Yes, people do that. I can give you the names of two good sperm banks—one in California and one in Virginia."

"Do they have pictures?" I asked.

"Only childhood photos. There is one other facility that provides adult photos, but we don't think that they provide the same sperm quality."

"Could we have their name anyway too?" I asked.

"Sure. I think you both need to go slow with this news, and really consider how you feel about it," said the counselor.

"Victoria is in a rush," said Gabriel.

I knew he was making a dig at me from our car conversation, but I ignored the barb. I explained to the psychologist, "Well, we have to decide about using our current egg donor because we're supposed to sign the contract now and begin soon."

I did not discuss anything further with Gabriel on the drive home. There was no point until we obtained more information. Plus we were both still upset with each other.

The next day I had to drive back to the New Jersey facility. My hysterosalpingogram, the test with the pink dye, was outdated by one month. Instead of a new pink dye procedure, I was getting something else this time—a saline sonogram.

The doctor arrived and said, "I know you. Do you remember me?"

He looked familiar. I stared at his goatee. Then I knew.

"Yes. You're the doctor from the first hospital that I used. You were the fellow."

"Now I'm working here."

The doctor explained that for this procedure he would place a balloon filled with saline solution inside me. Unfortunately, the water seeped out between my legs instead of emptying into my uterus. He had the nurse pump more water into the balloon with a catheter.

"Sorry about this. Medicine is not exact. It takes a little creativity. Your uterus has a marked downward tilt. I think the balloon will work this time. Otherwise we'll have to clamp the uterus shut to keep the balloon in, and you'll probably have cramping." Luckily it finally worked, and the doctor reported that my lining was good.

As I was leaving the clinic, my cell phone rang. It was Gabriel.

"Victoria, I have the results."

"What is it?"

"Not good."

"Oh, no."

"There was nothing. They found nothing again."

"Oh, God. Gabriel. I'm sorry. Then it must be a true finding."

"I'm not feeling very good about this. I have to go because I have a lot of patients waiting to see me."

"Gabriel, can I tell my family? I need to talk about it when I drive the next hour and a half home."

"Okay, but we'll talk more tonight."

I couldn't believe it. We needed a real miracle for Gabriel to get his sperm back.

First I called my parents. They had called me earlier from the airport. They were getting ready to board a plane to Florida for their winter stay. They didn't answer. They were probably in flight.

Next I called my brother.

"Mark, it's Victoria. Do you have a minute?"

"Yes. What's up?"

"I have crazy news."

"What?"

"Gabriel doesn't have sperm anymore."

"How can he not have sperm?"

"I don't know. He always had them before but now he doesn't."

"You should go see someone to find out what he has to do to get them back."

"We have a doctor's appointment next week, but I'm not sure if he can get them back."

"What will you do then?"

"I don't know. Gabriel brought up using a sperm donation from a cousin on his father's side."

"What are you going to do, ring his doorbell and ask for his sperm? Does Gabriel even know his cousins?"

"Some of them were at the wedding but some didn't come."

"Well, don't ask those."

"Maybe he'll use a stranger's sperm."

"He'll never do that," said Mark.

"Why do you say that?"

"Because his whole thing is continuing his family line. He grew up hearing about his ancestor. His mother probably still talks about him."

"She was going to put on Gabriel's father's tombstone that he's the seventh-generation male descendant."

"That's your answer. Plus the fact that he wants sperm from his father's relatives tells you something. This sperm dilemma will reveal the truth about his real motivations for having a baby and put him to the test."

"I'm not sure what he'll do."

"Did you tell Mom and Dad about this?"

"No, they're on the plane, I think."

"They'll tell you to do whatever you and Gabriel decide."

"Hold on, it's the call-waiting." I answered the other line. It was my parents. "It's them," I told Mark. "They must have just landed. I'll call you back later."

"Mom, hi. I was talking to Mark. Did you get in okay?"

"Yes, we're in a taxi going home."

"Can you talk for a minute?"

"Yes."

"I have new information about the baby."

"What?"

"We might not be able to use Gabriel's sperm. Right now he doesn't have any."

"What do you mean?"

"Two times, tests showed that he doesn't have sperm any more."

"Are you sure? Victoria just told me Gabriel has no sperm," she added for my father's benefit.

"Yes, I'm sure, and it might not be correctable."

"I'm really sorry to hear it. But maybe it just wasn't meant to be. You've tried all these times and it's enough."

"Maybe he'll want to use a donor sperm."

"What! Honey, she just said they may want to use a donor sperm. Let me put your father on."

"Victoria, that's crazy. Why would you want to do that? If he can't have his own child, there's no point," said my father.

My mother returned to the phone. "Victoria, it's time to put your foot down. Even if Gabriel wants to have a child that way, you tell him no. You don't want to be in your sixties like me with a teenager. The whole rest of your life would be devoted to raising a child. I don't know how long I have to live, and you won't know either once you're in your sixties."

"We'll see, Mom. I'll have to talk it over with Gabriel."

My brother had been wrong. My parents were not neutral. Gabriel and I would have to decide for ourselves.

That night Gabriel and I went to the local Irish pub. You could sit in a private booth. There was a long wooden table, wooden benches, and a wood wall to separate us from everyone else. They did not require a large party to fill the booth, and when it was available we could always get it.

"Gabriel, I can't believe this. There probably really is no sperm."

"I would have been back from work sooner, but I went on the internet. I was looking for an enzyme that might cause sperm deficiency. I bet I'm just missing one enzyme."

"Did you find any?"

"No. They don't have the technology yet."

"You sound like me looking in the *New York Times* for a breakthrough discovery that will let me use my own eggs. Miracle sperm-grow."

"I know."

"You're also in my position about whether to have the baby. Originally I told you I'd only use my own eggs. But this process changes you, and I agreed to use donor eggs because it was the only way we could get an IVF baby."

"I agree that you end up changed. I've been seriously considering using a donor sperm. I still want a child to raise from the beginning and to teach my values, even if it is not biologically mine."

"It's great to hear you say that," I answered.

Gabriel took my hand.

I went on, trying to make him feel better. "It's like we're in that O. Henry story, 'The Gift of the Magi.' The one where she cuts her hair to buy him a pocket watch chain, and he sells his watch to buy her combs for her hair. They both end up with losses but they are bound by each other's love and sacrifices. We may both give up our genes, but we'll gain a child to love and have our love for each other."

I felt close to Gabriel. The fact that he was willing to forgo his genes too meant a lot to me.

A week later Gabriel and I were both having difficulty sleeping. The next day we would be meeting with the male infertility specialist to find out more about Gabriel's sperm problem.

"Victoria, do you still love me?"

"Of course I love you."

"But I don't have any sperm."

"I have old eggs that don't work any more."

"But that's normal. Your eggs are supposed to age. You're not supposed to lose your sperm."

"I still love you."

The next day I met Gabriel at the hospital. Gabriel arrived first. I was directed into an examining room where he was waiting to see the doctor. Gabriel was sitting on a table. The top part of his body looked very business-like with a pale blue shirt, navy blue suit jacket, and coordinating maroon tie. The bottom part of him had a white electric blanket draped over his groin with his legs poking out. Gabriel explained that the blanket was to keep his testes warm. The doctor wanted to make sure that they didn't retract from the cold and hinder his upcoming exam.

The doctor arrived and shook our hands. He was a fit, athletic man. He quickly proceeded to feel Gabriel's testicles.

"There are no obstructions. You can get dressed and meet me in my office."

Gabriel and I walked to the doctor's office where he was already sitting behind his desk. Gabriel and I sat across from him in matching brown leather chairs.

"What is the problem?" asked Gabriel.

"It may just be an anomaly. We had a medical student who donated sperm one hundred times. Two times he had a count of zero and then it was normal again. The student may just have been under stress those two times."

"Then I may have sperm again when I donate for our next IVF cycle?"

"Yes. In fact I'd recommend giving sperm once and then if there is nothing there, do it again as soon as you are able. Sometimes only the second sample has sperm."

"We are using a donor egg this time," I explained.

"How old are you?" he asked.

"I'm forty-seven."

"That's good that you're using a donor egg. Out of over twenty thousand IVF trials, we have never found anyone over age forty-six who became pregnant with her own egg. Even at forty-six the chances are only three in a thousand."

His statistics seemed to prove that all of those older celebrities had used donor eggs.

"What about a sperm biopsy from the testes if we need it?" asked Gabriel.

"The biopsy with a needle to extract sperm works if there's a blockage. You don't have a blockage. You would require an operation under anesthesia. We would crack the testes open like an egg and look for sperm in the vesicles. Any sperm we might find would be only half as effective as ejaculated sperm. Also you might have permanent damage to your hormones."

"Would he still be able to have sex?" I asked.

"Yes, he could still perform fine, but he might lose his sexual desire if his testosterone level went way down. Then we'd have to give him replacement testosterone treatments. You'll probably get your sperm back naturally anyway, but if not, I see that you had a frozen sample when you did an IVF trial at our hospital three years ago."

"You mean he has frozen sperm? That's great," I said.

"The chances with frozen sperm are the same as with live sperm. In fact we thawed some of his sperm at the time to test them. They survived the thawing process and were good quality. We want to pick sperm with a moving tail. Then we know that they are alive. The dead ones don't move. Even a slight flutter tells you that it's living. Then the tail has to be immobilized so that it doesn't destroy the egg once we place the sperm inside," explained the doctor.

"I may not have frozen sperm anymore. I'm not sure if I paid the last bill. After three years I didn't think I needed them anymore," said Gabriel.

"They're not allowed to discard your sperm without notifying you in writing even if you're behind in your storage payments. Did you move?"

"No."

"Then they're probably there. I'll give you directions to the sperm office and you can check," said the doctor.

Gabriel and I walked to another building. We clicked the top of a silver bell, the type to call a store clerk, and waited for someone to appear. A woman emerged from behind glass doors.

"Do you have my sperm?" inquired Gabriel.

The nurse took his name and date of donation and went to look. She returned with a sheet of paper.

I had expected her to actually be carrying the sperm. Maybe she would have found it on the back shelves with the other merchandise that hadn't moved in the past few years.

She pointed to the paper and said, "Our records show you have two vials of sperm here from three years ago."

"Are they still good?" asked Gabriel.

"Honey, those sperm will outlast you and me. We could all be dead, and the sperm will be good forever."

"How do we get them to New Jersey?" asked Gabriel.

"You just have to fill out a shipping form. Let me know when the pickup will be. We don't like to have pickups on Fridays in case something goes wrong and the sperm are stranded over the weekend when we're closed."

Gabriel and I prepaid the shipping fee and left.

"Gabriel, we are so lucky. Your sperm got resurrected!"

"Even if I do have fresh sperm again, I want to use the frozen ones. They have been thawed and tested tried and true."

"Do you think we still should have a backup donor sperm?"

"No. We have two frozen vials and probably more live ones on the way."

Our sperm saga had a happy ending. That is, as long as the delivery truck didn't crash and smash Gabriel's sperm to smithereens.

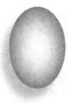

Nutcracker for the Infertile

E ven after the bad sperm episode, I had another egg donor dream. In this one I was watching a ten-year-old donor egg child who appeared on *60 Minutes* to talk about a film she was making about her donor egg life. All the while I watched the program I hoped my egg donor child would not go on TV to talk about her donor egg origin—I wanted to be her "true" mother and have the donor egg part fade into the background.

The morning before this dream, I had read an article on the front page of the *New York Times* about donor sperm half-siblings locating each other. The headline proclaimed, "Hello, I'm Your Sister. Our Father Is Donor 150." Apparently a website existed to help children find "lost" biological half-brothers and -sisters who came from the same donor sperm line. One child had instantly obtained twelve half-siblings spread across eight different mothers, although none could find out the identity of their sperm donor father since he had maintained anonymity. Another group of recently discovered half-siblings attended the choir concert of their teenage sperm line brother. I already knew that my Cinderella donor had already provided the eggs for two children who would be my baby's "blood" relatives. I didn't like the idea of my future baby's half-siblings coming to ring the doorbell and laying claim to my child.

Another concern was the chance that one day my child might meet and fall in love with one of his or her half-siblings. What if they had committed incest and discovered it years later, after they were married with children!

Most of the time, though, I dismissed such worries. In a month I was scheduled to proceed with the egg donation. At the New Jersey clinic, prospective donor egg mothers over the age of forty-four like me had to be cleared of any sign of bodily decay. I passed with flying colors.

Gabriel spoke with the New Jersey doctor about his consultation with the male infertility specialist. The New Jersey physician agreed that Gabriel would probably get his sperm back—it was like have a "bad-hair day." Gabriel told the doctor that he had paid to have his frozen sperm delivered to their facility. The Jersey doctor advocated that Gabriel rent a container of liquid nitrogen, like the sperm crock-pot that had arrived at our door, and drive the sperm over himself. It was too risky with the holiday mail.

That afternoon the phone rang. It was the nurse from our first facility, announcing that they had found a new donor for me. It had taken them more than a year and a half to find me one donor, and now within three weeks they'd found me two! This time the hospital had responded to my concern that the first donor might not be that intelligent: this donor was obtaining an undergraduate degree in the sciences and planned to pursue a master's degree as well. She was half Jewish, on her mother's side, so she would count as a "full-fledged Jew" by religious standards that mandated the maternal line be Jewish. Again I was surprised the hospital had given me another Jewish donor. I turned this donor down because I was too far along with the Cinderella donor. Luckily, I would keep my place on the waitlist in case something went wrong.

The next requirement from my New Jersey clinic was a phone consultation with their geneticist about my husband's genes and those of the donor. Mine were irrelevant. Neither my husband nor my donor were secret carriers of rare degenerative disorders, she informed me. The geneticist also promoted the genetic "improvement" provided by using the donor egg. With my genes and age, the chances would have been one in 16 for Downs syndrome, one in 11 for a chromosome disorder. The odds with the donor's egg decreased to less than one in 1,000 for Downs syndrome and one in 500 for chromosome disorders.

Finally the geneticist announced, "It's time for the most important information—the blood type. Do you know your blood type?"

"No. I haven't needed to know."

"You are type B+ and your husband is type A+. The critical piece of information is that the donor is O+. That means she and your husband could have either a type A baby like your husband or a type O. A baby with type O blood could have been your own baby. But there's a 50 percent chance it could turn out to be type A. Do you still want to use this donor?"

"Why wouldn't I want to?"

"For many recipients the blood type is a critical question. They'll only take a donor who will yield a baby with a blood type compatible with their own."

"Why?"

"Because they never plan to tell the baby that it came from a donor egg."

"I plan to tell the child its origin, so I guess I don't have to worry about the blood type dilemma."

I had never thought of the blood type as another critical factor in the donor selection process. I guess that donor egg recipient mothers didn't want a soap opera scene in the hospital, where the adult child would come to donate blood to his or her unconscious mother, and the doctor would exclaim, "You can't be her child and she can't be your mother. The blood type is wrong!"

Meanwhile it was nearly Christmas, and for the holidays Gabriel and I had decided to respond to a mailing about a new Off-Broadway production, *Infertility: The Musical That's Hard to Conceive.* I envisioned a singing sperm and egg, but when we arrived at the dinner theater, it proved to be an amusing psychological drama written by a couple who had infertility treatments. There were couples at every table, the majority of them same-sex. Of course, I realized: same-sex couples who wanted a child would *have* to make fertility decisions.

None of the main characters in the play had succeeded in their first fertility attempts, and all had moments when they had fantasies of perpetually screaming babies and thought of walking away. The married couple in the play wanted to join a motorcycle gang, the lesbians considered flying to the Caribbean, and the single woman planned to blow her money on a shopping spree. All of them decided to keep on trying anyway, but there was no happy ending: the play did not reveal in the end if they succeeded or not. Anyone who had tackled IVF could identify with the uncertainty and anxiety depicted. The fact that an Off-Broadway infertility play was showing to a full house reminded us that our situation was not so unusual. Gabriel and I were not alone.

Our donor needed to have her one-day evaluation before we could proceed. She wasn't available to come until after her final exams. Then one week later she would need to fly out again in order to be back in time for her first day of class.

Our New Jersey clinic was not happy with the scheduling restrictions of our donor. To meet her timing I would need to begin my Lupron shots in Florida before she was officially approved as a donor. If she flunked the psychological part during her one-day evaluation or one of her blood tests came back tainted, the whole cycle would need to be canceled. I told the clinic that I was willing to take the risk. I'd come this far with my donor, and I'd stick by her.

The night before the donor was to fly out for her one-day evaluation, the agency called. "Victoria, I have horrible news. The donor's teenage sister was in a car accident."

"Is she okay?"

"No, she's in a coma. A drunk driver hit her."

"Oh, my God. I'm really sorry."

"I'll keep you informed. Naturally the donor can't come tomorrow."

I felt terrible for the donor. Each day the agent called to give me an update. It was as if my own sibling was in a coma. I thought: if the donor comes and her sister doesn't make it, I'll name the baby after her sister. Gabriel was involved too. Every day at work he went online and looked up the local paper in the donor's small western town, searching for headlines about the donor's teenage sister. He never found any.

Finally the agent called with good news.

"She woke up from her coma!"

"That's great!"

"Most of her bones were broken, but she'll be okay."

"That's wonderful."

"The donor still wants to come."

"Are you sure?"

"Yes, she'll take the next available spot for her one-day evaluation."

I was happy that it had turned out well, but we weren't out of the woods yet. The agent called to tell me that she was concerned that the donor would score as "a mess" on all the psychological testing. The facility's psychologist reassured her that they would take into account the trauma of her sister's accident and not automatically rate her as "unstable" or "depressed." The agent also spoke with the doctor, who told her that, medically, the eggs should still be the same. I was worried that if my California doctor thought a college test made my first donor's eggs blacken, then this donor's eggs should be burnt to a crisp.

But then I received more bad news. I had continued to e-mail the woman I had met from the "gestational reduction" internet chat room. Her donation, from the woman with the red hair, had proceeded quickly, and my e-mail pal became pregnant. She was worried every day that she would lose the baby. Once she passed the three-month period, after which miscarriages were less likely, she was at last able to believe in the existence of her child.

She called me two weeks into the second trimester. "Victoria, I lost the baby."

"But you're beyond three months."

"I know, but it didn't matter. I had to give birth to the dead baby."

"What happened?"

"It wasn't growing properly, and they found out the brain was out of the skull."

"What? I never heard of such a thing."

"It was terrible."

"Didn't they pick it up on the sonogram?"

"No. They weren't looking for that. Plus we spent fifty thousand dollars."

"I'm really sorry. Do you know what you'll do now?"

"We'll adopt. I'm never going through that again."

"For a while it will still be awful, but once you have the adopted baby, it will feel like the one that was meant to be." I couldn't think of anything else to say to comfort her.

Her story disturbed me greatly. I might have used the same donor. It made me think of Chaucer's *Canterbury Tales*. I had read the book in college. The main characters, medieval pilgrims on the way to Canterbury, were allegorical representations of different vices. What if Gabriel and I also had sinned on our pilgrimage for a baby? Maybe Gabriel represented the sin of pride for trying to continue his famous bloodline. His punishment: losing the very sperm that was necessary to continue his line. My sin would be vanity. Rather than focusing simply on the creation of a baby, I had insisted on my own genetics, and when I had finally agreed to use a donor, I was punished for my narcissism by having the eggs of one donor wilting on the follicle and the sister of the other donor entering into a coma.

Most bothersome were worries about the baby that finally emerged from all these trials. What if in the end I actually gave birth to an infant with no brain? I would have to care for him every day. The children would never learn to love the new baby, and they'd be resentful of the hourly care I needed to lavish on their non-functional sibling. My parents would say, "I told you so," because they had thought that at my age I should never have started on the baby path. It took all my faith to believe that there would be baby redemption at the end of my journey.

On the fourth night of Chanukah, the Miracle of Lights, I experienced my own miracle. The children had returned from visiting with their father during the first half of our Florida vacation. We had missed lighting the other candles with them because this year Chanukah began on December twenty-fifth, and they were celebrating Christmas with their father's family.

After we lit the candles and sang "O Chanukah, O Chanukah, come light the menorah," Elizabeth announced that she had a present for me.

I unwrapped the gift—a book called *50,001+ Best Baby Names.*

"Thank you, Elizabeth, that's a wonderful present."

"I wanted to give you something to show that I support you in trying to have a baby. I'm behind you."

"That means a lot to me." I gave Elizabeth a big hug.

This was my miracle. Independently Elizabeth had voiced support for our baby attempts, and she didn't have to meet the baby first to be won over! She didn't know about the donor egg, I wouldn't tell her unless I was successful, and she might not be ready to accept that possibility. But at least she was open to the idea of a baby. Elizabeth had grown over the years. Originally she had been troubled after her family dissolved in divorce. Gradually she was becoming more comfortable with herself and her reconfigured family. She even could conceive of an additional family member without being threatened. I was proud of her!

While we were still on our Florida vacation, Gabriel made an appointment to meet with my parents' financial advisor. They highly recommended him. Gabriel wanted me to come too.

"Gabriel, why do you want to meet with a financial advisor?"

"It will be helpful."

"You can go. I'll sit by the pool. This is our vacation."

"I want to set up a financial plan to send our one or two babies to college."

"All right. I'll go with you."

I realized that Gabriel was very hopeful about this baby attempt. The last time he believed it was really going to work was when I had my first IVF cycle, and Gabriel was searching for a good pediatrician and obstetrician. Our chances were much higher with a donor egg, so maybe it really would happen this time.

When I was waiting for the taxi to take us to the airport for our return flight to New York, the cell phone rang. It was the nurse from my New Jersey clinic.

"I have bad news."

I was so used to bad news that I felt no emotional reaction. "What is it?"

"Your cycle is canceled—discontinue the medication."

"Why?"

"Your donor did not pass the screening."

"What did she fail?"

"I'm not at liberty to say. I can say that it was something medical. She passed the psychological. In fact I met her. She's quite lovely."

"Is it possible she'll clear in the future?"

"Perhaps. We'll know in a month. Meanwhile you and she need to stop your Lupron and just take birth control pills."

I didn't think I was ever going to find any eggs. I felt like the bird in the Dr. Seuss story that asked everyone, "Are you my mother?" Only I was asking, "Are you my donor egg mother?" But so far my story was the Grimms' fairy tale version, because all of my egg donors became cursed.

Two days later I was offered my third donor from the hospital waitlist. This one was Scandinavian and had no Jewish ancestry. Her information contained nothing objectionable and her special interests included "working out." I declined her too. I had decided to wait a month to see if my agency donor overcame her medical difficulty. If she was eliminated, then I might consider the hospital donor. The hospital's donors were already prescreened for all physical and psychological requirements. I would keep myself on the hospital waitlist, although eventually they might get annoyed if I kept turning down the donors they proposed.

Lisette and I went to the city the following Saturday to shop for her bat mitzvah dress. Lisette liked to be original. She did not want to buy her outfit from the store everyone from her school went to— the one at which Elizabeth had bought the same dress as another bat mitzvah girl. Lisette's sense of style had begun at a very young age. In fact she liked to "dress me," and her favorite show was *Project Runway*.

We were successful and found her an original dress. Meanwhile, on the train ride home, she leafed through the pages of *Teen Vogue*.

Then Lisette said, "Mom, I want to do that."

"Do what, Lisette?"

"Sell my eggs."

"What?"

"It says here that one girl got five thousand dollars for her eggs and another girl got ten thousand. I don't need all my eggs anyway."

"Lisette, you're too young for that."

I did not tell Lisette that I myself was buying someone else's eggs to create a new sibling for her. I was surprised that egg donation already had filtered down into the teen culture. I had mixed feelings about Elizabeth and Lisette ever donating their eggs. It would be a worthwhile return gesture, since someone else would have already donated to their mother. However, I would worry about their safety and their own future baby making ability. Indeed, the article described a "Lupron casualty" who had gone into a coma for months after donating her eggs. I would also be concerned that Elizabeth and Lisette might be in high demand, become addicted to donating, and never have to work. Two donations a year would pay their rent and living expenses.

The next day Gabriel went to New Jersey to help his mother. Elizabeth was in her room studying. Lisette and I had a free winter afternoon. We decided to surf the cable movies. Lisette found a new listing, *March of the Penguins*, and ordered it.

I envisioned cute little penguins waddling around the ice. Instead I watched a harrowing tale of the struggle of a penguin mother to give birth. First the penguins trekked up seventy miles to the nesting grounds. Then, once the mother laid one egg, she transferred it from her feet to the father's feet. He would have to spend months with no food balancing the egg on top of his feet and keeping it warm during blizzards. When the baby hatched, father and child had to wait for the mother, who marched the seventy miles back to the swimming hole where she would stock up on fish and dodge the seals waiting to eat her. Once she returned, the baby went back onto her feet, and she fed him regurgitated fish. Next it was the father's turn to hike the long distance back to water. In this way the parents devoted nine months to caring for the baby in this manner until it finally could go off on its own. I identified with the penguins and their birthing obstacles.

Three days later, thanks to Gabriel, we were all going to a Rolling Stones concert at Madison Square Garden. Elizabeth had been to concerts with her friends. I hadn't been to any in years and this was Lisette's first. When the Stones made their entrance and began playing "Jumpin' Jack Flash," I felt a rush of adrenaline, as if I were time-traveling back to my youth. The next song, "Let's Spend the Night Together," also catapulted me back to the past. The Stones were still rocking. Mick Jagger was a phenomenal performer. It was hard to believe that he was in his sixties. I realized that if I had a third child, we would not be able to take that one to the Stones. I didn't think that even Mick Jagger would be prancing around in his eighties.

Gabriel was also transformed by the music. He held my hand and bopped his head up and down as if he were stoned. Or maybe he was affected by the pot that fans near us were smoking.

Elizabeth was enjoying the concert. When we brought her to Broadway musicals, she pulled her iPod out of her pocket and listened to her own music, but not here. Lisette, however, who was always mesmerized by Broadway, hated the loud noise and flashing lights and now she wanted to go home.

The following evening at my book club, we toasted the sister of one of the book club members who also occasionally attended and was there that night. A single mother, she was due to deliver her daughter in three weeks. She told us that she had chosen the father from a Virginia sperm bank with only two criteria: height and weight. She was short and tended to overweight, so she had chosen the tallest and thinnest sperm donor that she could find. I didn't confide that I had almost used a sperm donor too, or that I was waiting to hear about the health status of my donor egg.

The next morning I read another *New York Times* article about donor sperm and eggs. There was a movement to pass a law that required revealing to children the identity of their sperm donor fathers and egg donor mothers. In New Zealand it was already illegal to keep the identity hidden, and in Great Britain children could get access to a donor's identity at age eighteen. Soon the forty thousand donor children born each year in the United States might clamor to know the identity of their parent donor. I hoped that in the future the United States would not demand unmasking the identity of egg donors. I didn't want the donor to become part of our family. I also hoped that my child would not yearn for a second mother. I still didn't want to share my child. The article also pointed out that someone could advertise as a non-smoking Ph.D. and really be a chain-smoking high school graduate. I agreed that there should be greater regulations of the qualifications of the donor.

That day we learned that Eve had survived her sixth cancer. Her three-month follow-up showed that her lung cancer had been obliterated by the radio wave zapping. Now she'd be able to attend Lisette's bat mitzvah in two months.

Later the clinic called. My donor had just passed the test she had failed earlier! The donation would proceed.

This donor had really proved herself. She had come for an evaluation when her sister was awake from her coma but still in the hospital. She had also agreed to donate even though it would no longer be during the dates of her college break.

Meanwhile I too had been tested. I had waited patiently for her eggs through a coma, health crisis, and my husband's sperm lapse. I had waited over three years for the creation of my baby. Now, at last, I'd know the result. All of the donor's strength in the face of adversity and all of my patience did not guarantee success. The donor could not affect the quality of her egg crop. She could not make her eggs manufacture a pregnancy for me as they had for her previous two couples. I could not make one of her eggs stick to my womb. We had no control—fate would decide.

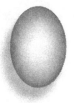

Start Spreading the News

My anxiety was skyrocketing. The end result of three and a half years of trying and over seventy thousand dollars spent would be determined with one flick of the urine stick. During the wait I resumed my biggest distraction: house hunting. The upgrade to an additional bedroom was astronomical in our neighborhood. Plus, with our IVF and bat mitzvah debts, we were no longer Grade A mortgage contenders.

House hunting was the only aspect of my IVF trials that Lisette enjoyed. She eagerly combed the newspapers for me and located cheap listings. She uncovered a four-bedroom house for sale by owner that was a steal. We drove by the house, expecting to find it next to a garbage dump or under a train track. We were pleasantly surprised to find it was an adorable cottage set back from the road. What was the catch? I wondered.

Lisette and I decided to check it out before the rest of the family. Elizabeth would be interested in staking out the largest bedroom, but only once we'd bought the house. And if it was worthwhile, we'd return with Gabriel on the weekend.

The next day Lisette and I arrived for our appointment at the cottage in the woods. The doorbell was answered by a boy who came up to Lisette's shoulder. When I looked closely at his face, I realized he was a grown man. A woman came to join him. She was even smaller. They were a dwarf couple.

They proudly took Lisette and me on a tour of their home. The kitchen had been custom designed. The sink and stove were the proper height for the dress-up corner of a kindergarten classroom. The table and chairs were a good size for Goldilocks in preschool. The updated bathrooms had the same low to the ground toilets used by the local nursery school. Lisette and I had to bend down to enter the bedroom doorways. The house would have been a perfect playhouse for my yet unborn child, but the rest of us, even Lisette, were too big for it.

The drawback to the next house was clear from the start: it had only two bedrooms. Our entire reason for moving would be to obtain a fourth bedroom. Still a realtor told me about this house and insisted it was not to be missed. Once again Lisette and I were the preliminary scouting party. At the last moment Elizabeth came too. She had been at the house for Halloween trick-or-treating and reported that it was incredible. We all fell in love with it. The living room was even more dramatic than ours. There were fourteen-foot ceilings, wooden beams, a balcony, mosaic floor tiles, and wrought iron grill work. The den was paneled, and there were fireplaces in three rooms. I told Gabriel about the house.

"Gabriel, we all saw a house that's worth looking at."

"What's it like?"

"It has a fantastic living room, a paneled den, a real eat-in kitchen, and a yard."

"How many bedrooms?"

"That's the catch."

"Victoria, we need four. If it only has three again, what's the point of moving?"

"Well, actually, it only has two."

"What? Don't be ridiculous. You're wasting your time."

"It's better than it sounds. There are really more rooms then you think. Just come see it."

"All right, but we're going to be in and out fast."

We spent an hour and a half in the house. Even practical Gabriel was charmed by the living room. I explained my bedroom approach. We could sleep in the large den downstairs and the baby would be in a bassinette with us for the first six months. Then the baby could move upstairs to the dressing room that was attached to the master bedroom. Elizabeth could sleep in the master and Lisette in the smaller bedroom. By utilizing the den and the dressing room, we could transform a two-bedroom house into a four-bedroom one. Of course if there were twins, we'd have a problem.

Gabriel could see the possibilities of my bedroom arrangements (I'd had previous practice when I squeezed four people into my Junior Four apartment). The house appealed to him, and he decided to make a low offer. That way even if there was no baby we could make a house trade and upgrade. The owners of the house were not overwhelmed by gratitude. They refused even to counter-offer. Gabriel said we could wait.

Despite the diversion of house hunting, my anxiety level was still high. If this didn't work, we'd finally hit the baby brick wall. What if Gabriel dumped me for a younger, fertile woman? I always thought that he wouldn't be like Henry VIII or Napoleon, but maybe he would.

At our temple we all attended the Friday night service together. Lisette needed to go five times before her bat mitzvah. This service was particularly moving because a single woman in her twenties had decided on her own to convert to Judaism that night. Three hundred years ago her family had been Jewish, but they had intermarried in South Carolina and became Catholics. Now she was reclaiming her roots. Her enthusiasm for Judaism made me feel that I was taking my religion of birth for granted. She was very pretty. One of the older Jewish congregants joked that he would have to find her a nice Jewish boy. I noticed Gabriel staring at her. I thought again about what had happened with Pierre. After I discovered Pierre's married paramour, I also learned about his liaison with our former housekeeper. She apologized to me in the parking lot of our grocery store, even telling me that at the time they were involved, Pierre's married mistress flew in from California to tell her to leave "her man" alone. What if Gabriel's eyeing of the new Jewish convert progressed further? What if he ran off with her once I failed to bear him a child? Then I told myself that he was committed to me, and that, if need be, we would bear the loss of our child together.

For my third monitoring I went to the clinic in New York; New

Jersey was too far to make the 6:30 a.m. monitoring there. I was worried, because four days earlier my uterine lining had been rated a six, which was too thin: it was supposed to be a seven or above. Fortunately, the tests at the clinic showed that my lining had progressed to a twelve. This IVF cycle was different because the only part of me I could cheer for was my uterine lining.

Elizabeth's movie was finally being released in theaters so we could view her on the big screen. In the meantime, she had asked to try modeling too. She was a fan of the TV show *America's Next Top Model*. The agent sent out pictures and soon she was requested by the Girl Scouts of America. Two weeks later, we learned that she had booked the photo shoot. She was ecstatic to have landed her first modeling job.

The nurse from the New Jersey clinic called. We had missed checking one box on the consent form. The transfer could not proceed until that page was completed and signed.

"Gabriel, we forgot to check off the page about what will happen to any frozen embryos if we get divorced. We need to fill it out immediately."

"Okay, we'll fill it out."

"We can just put that they should discard the embryos."

Gabriel was silent.

"Why do you want custody of them? So if we got divorced another woman could carry them for you?"

"Victoria, I may not have any more sperm."

"Fine. If you want custody of the eggs you can have them."

"That's okay. We can throw them out."

So I checked the discard box.

Apparently Gabriel wanted a backup plan as much as some of those young career women who were freezing their eggs.

Gabriel and I planned to tell the children we were using a donor egg if I became pregnant, but we hadn't decided exactly how or when. The question forced itself suddenly one afternoon when I was picking up Elizabeth from track practice, and Lisette called me from home on my cell phone.

"Mom, are you using a donor egg?" asked Lisette.

"Why are you asking that?"

"I heard someone leave a message about a donor."

"Maybe. I'll talk about it when I get home."

"No! Don't do that! Don't use a donor."

"I'll talk to you soon, Lisette."

I would not lie. Since Lisette had overheard about the donor, I would have to discuss it with her now. She would tell Elizabeth as soon as she walked through the door, so I also would have to explain it to Elizabeth. I called Gabriel at work to tell him that I would have to tell the children because Lisette had found out and was upset.

Elizabeth ran over to the car in her track shorts.

"Elizabeth, I have to tell you something important."

"What is it? Is it bad?"

"No. Everyone is fine. I wanted to tell you that this time your dad and I are trying for a baby with a donor egg."

Elizabeth's eyes widened.

"We're trying someone else's eggs because mine haven't worked."

"I've read about egg donors. It helps them pay for college."

"Well, they usually need the money."

"I'm okay with it, Mom."

"Are you sure?"

"Yes."

"I have pictures that you can see if you want. I chose someone who looks like you. She even likes the same sports."

"That's cool."

"I don't want you to tell your friends at this point. First we have to decide when we'll tell the baby. It wouldn't be fair if everyone at your school already knew that the baby came from a donor egg."

"All right."

"If you have any questions you can ask me whenever you want."

Gabriel called in on my cell, and I said that I had just given Elizabeth the news. I handed Elizabeth the phone, and he told her that he loved her. When we got home, Elizabeth asked to see photos of the donor. She thought that she was pretty. "She looks so young!" she said.

I answered, "Well, she is very young."

I played back the message on the machine. The nurse said that the donor was receiving her hCG that night. Two days later would come the retrieval. My husband would be needed that morning to give his sperm. Then, three to five days later, I'd go for the transfer.

After hearing the message, I searched for Lisette. She wasn't answering. I found her in her room.

"Lisette, I want to talk about what you heard on the machine about a donor."

"I'm not talking to you."

"We need to discuss it if you want to know what's going on."

"All right."

"Lisette, I was going to tell you about the donor if I became pregnant, but you didn't need to know about it yet."

"Mom, don't use a donor!"

"Do you even know what a donor is?"

"Yes, I know."

"I've tried five times with my egg and this is the only way that the doctors think that it could work."

"Mom, it'll be weird when someone else gives birth to the baby."

"Lisette, that's a surrogate. I'd be carrying the baby and delivering it. It would just be someone else's egg."

"That would be worse. It wouldn't be your genes. It would be some other person's family line. Something could be the matter with them. Plus the child would be really depressed. You wouldn't even be its mother. It would be confused about who its mother is. That's not fair. I know a girl who's depressed because she was adopted and won't ever know her real parents."

"Not everyone who is adopted is depressed. They can be happy too. We'd have to explain it to the child."

"You're too old to be a mother anyway. Forget about it."

"Lisette, you know I would still love you. You'd still be special to me."

"It's not that. You won't have any time. We won't be able to go on any vacations. Everyone will just care about the baby."

"I'd still have time for you. Your life would still be the same."

"My dad wants babies too. That's too many babies."

"His wife is younger. Maybe they'll wait a while." (Pierre had recently married a woman who was roughly half his age, half his weight, and twice as tall.)

"Who's going to walk the dog? Elizabeth and I never walk him. Only you do. No one will care about the dog."

"I'll still care for the dog, and I'll still care for you too."

"Well, maybe it will be okay—but only with your egg. You can't use anyone else's egg. I'll be really mad if you do."

I decided not to point out again that we already were using someone else's egg. Lisette had enough to handle. Her bat mitzvah was in two weeks, and she was juggling schoolwork and memorizing Hebrew prayers. If I really became pregnant, then some time, after the bat mitzvah, I'd revisit the topic. Of course, since Elizabeth fully understood and had even viewed photos of the donor, Lisette and I might have to face the subject again sooner.

Gabriel wanted to know whether sperm would turn up this time when he went to donate. It was a macho matter for him. I wasn't as concerned, since we now knew that the frozen backup sperm had been delivered safely.

Gabriel also hoped to see the donor in the waiting room. He was curious about the woman who would be the mother of his child. He looked at her photos again so he would recognize her. I warned him not to talk with her. I didn't want her to be able to identify him in the future.

Later, Gabriel called from the clinic. He had not found our donor, but he had successfully made his deposit. This third facility had an ample supply of magazines and videos. Sweetly, he confided that he had kissed my photo before and after, although he didn't elaborate about what he'd looked at in order to get aroused. Then he said he'd call again once they'd checked out the donation.

Gabriel rang back with good and bad news. The good news was that his sperm was back. The bad news was their quality was poor. The andrologist (sperm specialist) did not like their chemical consistency.

Gabriel would have to ejaculate one more time. He had no problem with that, but unfortunately the results were the same. It was time to thaw the frozen sperm. Gabriel was told to wait.

Soon he called again with an update. "Victoria, there's a problem with the sperm."

"Oh, God, what now?"

"They thawed, but they're not moving."

"You mean they're dead?"

"Well, they'll try to bring them back to life with a chemical. Otherwise they may do an emergency operation on me and try to locate better sperm."

I did not imagine that there was much chance of resurrecting dead sperm. I considered calling the agency to see if they had any backup sperm we could order immediately. In a desperate moment I even fantasized that, since it was an emergency, maybe one of the doctors at the clinic could go into the bathroom and donate his sperm. Otherwise the donor's forty-thousand-dollar golden eggs might be lying fallow on the lab table, with no way to fertilize them. What if they performed the search-and-remove operation on Gabriel and it wasn't successful? What if they cut something in his testicles by mistake, or he died from the anesthesia? Hadn't the doctor told us the procedure could result in loss of libido? I didn't want to sacrifice our sex life. I felt cornered. A great sadness started to rise within me. This would be my sixth failed IVF attempt—seventh if I counted the last one, when the previous donor's eggs stopped growing.

Gabriel called back. He sounded more animated.

"Is the news any better?"

"The sperm are moving! The chemical brought them back to life."

"Thank the Lord! We're back too!"

The following day, the nurse told me that the donor had produced forty-two eggs, of which twenty had fertilized. I felt a little jealous of the success my husband had had with another woman. But finally it might really work.

While waiting to find out if I would be a day-three or day-five transfer, I discovered new fertility reading material. This time there was a ten-page spread in the *New York Times Magazine* about donor sperm. Increasing numbers of single women were forgetting about finding Mr. Right and instead mail-ordering sperm. The women were choosy. No sperm bank could offer specimens from men under 5'9" because there were no buyers for shorter men's seed. Maybe one day single men would buy donor eggs for their progeny and forgo having wives altogether.

Even with a donor egg, it was still a day-three transfer. When I arrived at the clinic, I had to drink six glasses of water within one hour so that there would be fluid for my sonogram. I was asked if I wanted to participate in an acupuncture study. They would place needles all over my body for twenty-five minutes before and after the transfer. The side effects could be fainting, bleeding, pain, and bruises. I explained that I was "vasovagal" and would probably faint from all of the needles. The spokesperson for the procedure said it wouldn't be so bad once I got used to it and that it could be relaxing. I said maybe I'd try it some other time. The thought of all those needles made my anxiety soar. As for the egg transfer, I was a seasoned pro at that.

I was the fifth and last person scheduled for a transfer. The doctor handed me a computer picture of my donor's embryos. He explained that there was some fragmentation of the embryos and that I had the best chance with three particular ones. The doctor recommended transferring all three into my womb and said seven more were contenders for freezing if they developed well. In my earlier trials with my own eggs, I told him, my embryos were better. The "young genetics" of the donor still meant I had a greater chance of pregnancy with these embryos than with mine, he replied. He also explained that the odds for triplets were not great given the embryo quality, but that if needed I could reduce one with only a 5 to 8 percent chance of losing them all.

I agreed to transfer three. I would follow his advice. But I really didn't want triplets. For the sake of my health and the babies' I would most likely reduce. I worried that I would probably be forever haunted by the specter of the child that I had destroyed.

Next I followed the doctor into the operating room and lay down on the bed. The physician and his nursing assistant rubbed warm gel on my stomach and placed the arm of the sonogram machine on my stomach. The sonogram showed there wasn't enough fluid yet, and the doctor couldn't locate my uterus. The doctor left and the nurse brought me cups of water to gulp: it felt a little like a party drinking game. The doctor returned for another look, but there was still no sign of my uterus. He departed again, and gingerly the nurse wiped off the sonogram fluid, draped me again carefully with the medical cloths, and went for more water. I began to feel nauseated from all of the guzzling. I felt very alone. I was also was shivering with cold, and I wondered if this was ever going to work. There was a glass window in the wall of the adjacent embryology lab. I could see a man walking around and straightening the room. I hoped I was still covered and that he wasn't a voyeur. The nurse returned to see if she could locate my uterus. When it still failed to appear, she started sighing loudly. Probably otherwise she could have gone home by now. When the doctor returned, he could find part of my uterus, but not all of it.

He told the nurse, "We'll have to give her more water."

"But she's already had twenty cups."

"Eventually we'll get a good view."

By now it all felt like water torture. Acupuncture would have been preferable. This time when the nurse walked out of the room, she left the gel dripping on my stomach, my body uncovered, and the metal arm of the sonogram machine on my stomach. Maybe next she'd pull the gurney out from under me. I sure hoped they'd find my uterus soon.

The nurse returned first. She pressed hard on my abdomen with the sonogram locater, trying every angle until from the left side, applying extreme pressure, she finally found my entire uterus. "Don't move!" she yelled as she ran out of the room.

The doctor returned. She started bench-pressing me again.

"I had it before. Look, I got it!"

The doctor concurred. She was pressing down on me with as much gusto as a sumo wrestler. "By now, you probably want to report me for patient abuse." The nurse laughed.

I didn't think that it was funny. I also was worried that she would lose her chokehold at the critical moment and the embryos would be launched out of the catheter into empty space. The doctor explained that it was crucial to maintain visual contact. On the sonogram monitor screen he pointed out the tiny white light that were the embryos and the *X* that was the landing target. It was a kind of ovarian video game. I watched the light slowly travel toward the *X* and prayed for a hit. Luckily, the doctor scored.

Normally I would have waited twenty minutes with my legs up before going to the bathroom, but in my case the doctor and nursed joked that I would be in agony soon, and they determined that a bed pan was in order. Once I relieved myself, they told me my husband was in the waiting room, and I was free to go home.

I hugged Gabriel and suggested dinner at the romantic Victorian

Grade A Baby Eggs

restaurant we went to after one of the donor egg groups.

At dinner Gabriel became very quiet.

"What's wrong?"

"What if it doesn't work?"

"There might be frozen ones too."

"But if we fail, there's no baby. I'm starting to feel depressed. Yet I wouldn't want to put you through this again."

I thought it was kind of him to think about me. He knew that all of the hormones were torture enough. Plus it could damage my body.

Then he said, "We could always use a surrogate next time."

"What? Gabriel, we're not using a surrogate. This is supposed to be it."

"I just wish that the last time we had used a donor instead of your eggs. Then we could have tried twice with donor eggs."

"Gabriel, even if we use a donor one more time you don't have much frozen sperm left. Why are you focusing on the negative? You should be happy. We finally used a donor and it might work."

"I just don't want to get my hopes up and be left with nothing."

I hoped that it succeeded. I was a fighter, but I wasn't sure that I wanted to keep battling. I wanted closure. Either this should be our last try, or we could continue only if there were frozen embryos. I didn't think that I could handle an endless stream of internet donor choices, thrown-away money, and bereavement when the process failed. Plus I really wanted us to focus on each other, and on Lisette and Elizabeth. The quest for a baby had been overshadowing everything, including them.

A few days passed, and I had to keep waiting. It felt like the entrance to a special kind of monorail ride. I wanted to board and to begin the ride of raising another child, but I was also scared. Once I embarked there would be no getting off. I would be zooming along the monorail for the next eighteen years until my child entered college. I would not exit until age sixty-six. Meanwhile, on the eve of my forty-eighth birthday, AARP had sent me an invitation to join. When Gabriel and I retired, we'd have to tote our youngster with us to the retirement home.

My pregnancy blood test was scheduled for the day before Lisette's bat mitzvah. If I wasn't pregnant, Gabriel and I would have to push aside our loss and be happy for Lisette on her special day. If I was pregnant, it might be hard to hide it from the bat mitzvah girl. My friends would be asking me, and she might overhear the news. If people began hugging and congratulating us, she would guess that a new sibling must be on the way, and she would be miserable. My friend Star recommended that we delay taking the pregnancy test until the day after the bat mitzvah. I called the nurse, and she said that medically it would be fine to wait. Gabriel and I agreed to do just that.

This time I felt not even the slightest hint of nausea, not even after eating spicy food at night. I guessed that meant there was no pregnancy. Over and over my mind kept repeating the line from *Macbeth*, "full of sound and fury, signifying nothing." The mailman delivered a check from the hospital for a few thousand dollars. At first I was positive the refund meant no eggs had been frozen. When I called, I discovered it was because the donor and I had been monitored elsewhere. Luckily I was so busy with Lisette's bat mitzvah, attending to last-minute details such as buying snacks, cookies, and craft store souvenirs for the gift bags of the out-of-town hotel guests that I was able to stop myself from buying home pregnancy tests.

Lisette was wonderful during the Saturday bat mitzvah service. Her days of practicing Hebrew in the car and in the basement with the dog paid off. She presented her Torah and Haftarah portions with great poise.

The weather on Sunday for the party was fantastic, and for a brief moment the guests had great views of the blooming orchids in the gardens. Then, right after the cocktail hour, Lisette insisted on pulling down all the shades in the room to evoke the feeling of a nightclub. When Gabriel wasn't looking, I had a few sips of wine. If I wasn't pregnant, I didn't want to resent missing all of the alcohol at the open bar.

My plan was to dash to the drugstore as soon as the party ended and purchase a home pregnancy test for that night. Instead I ended up with my hands in the garbage for two hours. Lisette's shopping bag with all of the presents and scrapbooks made for her by her closest friends was missing. We searched through all the garbage bags before sending them to the compacter. Then we called the last party guests to see if anyone had taken the bag by mistake. No luck. Later that evening at home, we received a call that a staff member had put the bag into the safe but neglected to tell anyone. We were all relieved. It was too late to buy a pregnancy test, and I decided that we'd had enough excitement for the night.

The next morning I went to the local lab for the blood test. The lab technician remembered me. I told her that this was the sixth and probably last pregnancy attempt. If I failed, she suggested, I could aspire to be like Angelina Jolie and start adopting children from different continents. Afterward, I went to work. It would take great willpower to focus on my patients and not on the looming test result.

Just as I arrived at the office to see my Long Island patients, my cell phone rang. It was the nurse. She said that my pregnancy results had already come. "I wish that I had better news."

"You mean I'm not pregnant?"

"Yes. They usually do a follow-up blood test, but the hCG level was minus two. That's so low that there's no reason to do it."

"I can't believe there's nothing. Still, I shouldn't be surprised, because I wasn't feeling nauseated."

"I have more bad news."

"There's nothing frozen either?"

"That's right. You can make a follow-up appointment to speak with the doctor."

As soon as I hung up, Gabriel called. He had requested that the lab fax a copy of the result to his office, as well as to the New Jersey clinic. "Victoria, you can stop taking your medication."

"I know, they just called me. I'm so sorry, Gabriel. If you want, we can do it again."

"I've had enough."

"We can still decide. I'll do whatever you want."

I felt cheated. After all of these attempts I would go home with nothing. It was as if our baby had been kidnapped before it ever got born—for a moment I felt a panic, as if our actual child had been mysteriously abducted.

Unbelievably my first patient was arriving in fifteen minutes. I did not know how I would concentrate. I felt the urge to place a "went home for emergency" sign on the door. Instead I struggled to focus on a full caseload. As the afternoon progressed I felt more and more mournful. I only managed to survive the day by ignoring my baby thoughts.

Gabriel called at the end of the day. He suggested that we meet back in Westchester at the Indian restaurant with the elephant wall hangings.

As I was driving home, at the start of a rainstorm, my cell phone rang. It was my friend Star, who had come in from Florida for Lisette's bat mitzvah.

"Victoria, the bat mitzvah was wonderful. I had such a good time. You all looked great."

"We were so glad you could come."

"And?"

"Star, I'm not pregnant."

"I was positive you would tell me you were pregnant."

"No, there was no baby and no frozen eggs. There was nothing."

"I'm really sorry."

Throughout my drive in the pouring rain, the phone kept ringing with friends and relatives asking what happened. They all knew that I had delayed the blood test until after the bat mitzvah. It was hard telling everyone that we had not succeeded. Even with a donor egg, I had come up short. Gabriel and I had really expected this baby. We were left with a void. We had always maintained hope. The existence of the baby was real to us. Now it was snatched away. It seemed outrageous that all the fertility technology failed us. It also seemed ridiculous that we put so much time and money into a doomed baby. If I had known the outcome, I might not have done it at all. All those medications, operations, all that money and hope for a baby that never developed. But Gabriel and I had really needed to try. We had made that commitment together. We needed to fail in order to move forward. I couldn't accept the loss of my baby until I had done everything possible to obtain it. Gabriel had to go through it as well. We couldn't walk away with a sense of finality until we'd both struggled with the fertility process.

When I arrived at the restaurant, Gabriel was already there. I gave him a big hug. We asked for a private booth.

"Gabriel, I'm really sorry. If you want to try again with a donor egg, we can. We also could adopt if you want to be sure that we'll get a baby."

"My first instinct when I heard was to stop it here."

"Well, maybe it's too soon to know what we want."

"I'm feeling really depressed. I want you to get those two bears off of my night table." Gabriel was referring to the pink and blue baby bears in a carriage that he, Elizabeth, and Lisette had brought home for me when I had my chemical pregnancy. "Maybe it would be easier if I wasn't trying to continue my father's blood line."

"Even if we had a baby, the line could still end if there were no grandchildren."

"I know that."

"Even with the better donor odds, we weren't the lucky ones."

"My unmarried friends still have the possibility that one day they'll marry and have children. For me, the door will be closed forever."

"As they keep getting older, it's unlikely they'll find women thirty years younger who want to bear their children."

"It's just going to be really hard for me."

"I hope you don't want me to die so you can meet a younger woman," I joked morbidly.

"Of course not."

"We need to focus on Elizabeth and Lisette. They both love you."

"I know, but it would be nice to raise a child from the beginning. Plus they still have their dad too."

"You're the one living with them. He hardly ever visits."

"You may be right that we're getting too old to raise a child. It could ruin everyone's lifestyle, the children's as well as ours."

My cell phone rang. It was Elizabeth.

"Mom, are you pregnant?"

"No, I'm not."

"Oh, I'm sorry. I know you really tried," commiserated Elizabeth.

"It's okay. Put Lisette on the phone. I'd better tell her too."

"Lisette, I'm not pregnant."

"I'm sorry," she said in a happy, relieved voice.

When we arrived home, Elizabeth told Gabriel she was sorry. She said, "You still have Lisette and me."

"I know, and you have me too."

A bill was waiting for us from the agency. Apparently we owed them a lot more money. We had to pay for the canceled flight when the donor's sister had been in a coma, additional hotel bills, and the monitoring fees from her clinic in the Midwest, which charged higher rates than my New York hospitals. Every blood test was five hundred dollars. Gabriel said, "They definitely need legal regulations for donor eggs. This is a racket." We owed almost fifty thousand dollars for this last cycle alone.

Later that evening Gabriel emerged from his basement retreat and talked to me again.

"I have an idea."

"What?"

"Once I get money again, I'm going to start a scholarship fund in my father's name at his temple. Every year a child will have the ability to go to a Jewish camp."

"That's a great idea, Gabriel."

"I need to have a way to honor my father and to carry on his name."

"I'm sure he really would have appreciated it."

I was delighted that Gabriel was once again trying to be constructive. Maybe he would even recover from the loss of his own child.

"I'm also going to try to work less. I could take off some four-day weekends."

Our baby losses had made us take stock of our lives.

A few weeks later, I went out to lunch with a friend from my book club.

She said, "I heard you're looking for a four-bedroom house."

"We were, but we don't need it now. We were trying to have a baby with IVF, but it didn't work." Then I began sobbing.

"I'm sorry," she said.

I proceeded with my life activities, but my feeling of loss was set on a hairspring trigger.

Later that week I went to the mall with Lisette. During previous visits there I had still carried the hope of a new baby. This time I stared longingly at someone else's baby, knowing I would never have one with Gabriel. Lisette patted my arm and said "It's okay, Mom."

Another friend from my book club invited me to her house. She was babysitting for the infant her sister had recently delivered with the sperm donor. I declined the invitation. It would be too painful to spend a few hours holding the baby and thinking about how I never got mine.

When Gabriel and I arrived for our 7:30 a.m. feedback session with the doctor, it was difficult to enter the building. In the waiting room I gazed at the pretty fish swimming in the tank and sipped the free hot chocolate, but I was ready to burst into tears. The feeling of failure was overwhelming. I stared at all of the other hopeful couples who might bring home a baby. I knew now that I would never be one of them.

The doctor told us that we had just been unlucky. He recommended that we cycle again with the same egg donor or another one who produced a lot of eggs. Then we could try for a pregnancy as well as the backup of frozen eggs. He explained the embryos don't always keep dividing to the fifth day, when they can be frozen; ours had all discontinued growing at day three. He said not to worry. The fact that the remaining embryos stopped thriving did not mean that the transferred embryos had also stopped developing within me on day three, since they always do better inside the womb. The doctor suggested that we have repeated attempts with a donor. The odds increased with a younger egg, and if we kept trying, it should eventually work.

For us, the doctor's timing was off. Whereas Gabriel and I were looking for closure, the doctor was advocating a perpetual IVF loop. He said he was very sorry for our loss. He realized how hard it must be to try so many times and fail.

At the end of our appointment, the doctor reiterated that embryos not transferred into a woman's womb frequently don't survive beyond day three. He also remarked that there was a small possibility that the embryos had stopped growing in the Petrie dish because of a "sperm issue." He explained that research indicated that in the first few days, embryo development was directed by the genetics of the woman's egg, but that afterward the genetic contribution of the sperm was activated. Failure of the embryo to continue dividing could be pure chance, or it could be because the sperm had malfunctioned. The doctor suggested we create a controlled experiment with donor eggs, either from the same donor or from someone else with a high egg output. Then for our next attempt we could fertilize half of the eggs with Gabriel's sperm and the other half with a donor's sperm. The two groups of embryos could be observed. At day three the two best embryos from Gabriel and the two best embryos from the sperm donor would be implanted in my uterus. The remaining embryos would continue to be observed and compared.

This struck me as an elaborate means to learn more about Gabriel's sperm. If I became pregnant I wouldn't even know the father of my child. I suppose I could request DNA testing to determine the paternity.

I really wanted to have a child with Gabriel. I couldn't believe that after three and a half years we would have no infant. It was hard to relinquish our dream for a baby. Yet I also was relieved. No more shots, hormones, and emotional roller coasters.

I would still research fertility findings. Perhaps in the near future there would be a stem cell discovery that allowed me to use my own egg or a guaranteed method to make it succeed with a donor egg. In the meantime I would strive to live life to the fullest and to focus on those that I already loved rather than on the phantom baby that just could not be born.

Grade A Baby Eggs

Epilogue

Home Sweet Home—June 2006

W e didn't have our baby, but we did get our two-bedroom house. The owners came back to us a few months later. Sometimes life creates a detour. You run as hard as you can down one path and get thrown onto another.

We got the twist ending. When I was a young teen, I watched popular science fiction offerings on television such as *The Twilight Zone*, *The Outer Limits*, and *Night Gallery*. These programs specialized in a surprise, surrealistic finale. After my failure with IVF technology, I remembered a particular *Night Gallery* episode. It featured a man who regularly went to a museum and gazed at a tranquil painting of a rowboat floating in the water. He fantasized about sitting in the boat and longed to enter the picture. One day his wish came true. He was inside the painting! But the exhibition had been changed, and he had leapt into a different scene, in which he was being perpetually tortured.

I tried for years to catapult into the painting that depicted Gabriel and me holding our baby. This was our fantasy image. But that painting was no longer an option. It was up to me to decide which picture I created next. I realized I could lacerate myself mentally for not producing a baby and become trapped in overwhelming pain and sorrow. Instead I chose to paint a new picture. Gabriel, Elizabeth, Lisette, and I were happily settled into our new home. This was not the creation we had expected, but it was another way to cherish life together.

That August, my parents took Mark's family and ours on a cruise to Alaska to celebrate their upcoming fiftieth wedding anniversary. My mother was ecstatic to have everyone there. She planned group activities. We went on the dog-sledding excursion. Because there was no snow, we sat on a sled with wheels and were pulled around in circles on the grass by the dog team. Elizabeth, Lisette, and my nieces spent the rest of the time playing happily with three recently delivered, adorable puppies. At dinner my father discussed his being nominated for a national Lasker medical award because of his discovery of a lifesaving medical procedure. If he won it, he would have fulfilled his orphanage vow to make something of himself. (The following month, when someone else got it, he was at first devastated. Then the Lasker committee asked him to apply again for the following year. In the meantime, he would learn to accept his existing accomplishments without focusing on the award that he still might not win.) After dinner, we all went to the show. A drunk, slobbering man sat behind Mark's oldest daughter and whispered sweet nothings in her ear like "Shut up! You're talking too much" and "I don't like you." My niece started crying. Mark leaned over to the man and almost punched him. My mother intervened by hustling the family to the front row. Fortunately the drunken man didn't follow.

After the show, Gabriel and I went to the top deck to have a drink at the disco. We sat together on the love seat, looked out at the waves of the ocean and held hands as we sipped our daiquiris. The romantic moment was interrupted when we heard laughing from the other side of the room. There was Elizabeth, sitting next to a boy and having her own romantic interlude! Lisette, we knew, was hanging out with her cousins and would probably not appear with a male companion.

When the cruise was ending, Gabriel and I went to pick up the family photo we'd ordered of the four of us. Gabriel studied the picture carefully, then yelled, "Oh my God!"

"What is it?"

He pointed. I burst out laughing. There, coming out of Gabriel's pants, was what looked like an exposed, erect penis.

"Gabriel, how did that get there?"

"I don't know. I think it's the sleeve of my coat that I had tied around my waist."

"You look like a flasher."

We showed the photo to the attendant, who tried to maintain a straight face as he studied the situation. He thought it was correctable. Later that day, we picked up a new picture. On this it looked like the white finger of a glove had been slid over Gabriel's still erect "penis." I asked the photo technician if he could do any better. The final snapshot was a success. Gabriel's penis had been amputated and filled in with a color that matched the rest of his pants.

Now at last we were a "regular," intact family. We had bonded on the ship with extended and immediate family, and we had the photo to show it.

For the grand finale, Gabriel and I flew with the girls from Seattle, where the cruise ship docked, to San Francisco. We would return late that evening to Seattle. We walked around Ghirardelli Square and Fisherman's Wharf. Then we ate a wonderful meal while enjoying a view of Alcatraz across the water. Gabriel and Lisette wanted dessert. Elizabeth said, "There's no time. We'll miss the plane." Gabriel and Lisette enjoyed their ice cream sundaes. We strolled out of the restaurant, expecting to hail a cab as we always did in New York City. There were no taxis passing by Fisherman's Wharf. When we finally found one, it got us to the airline twenty-two minutes before takeoff. They hadn't boarded yet, but the airline had already given away our seats along with those of several other screaming, irate passengers. The airline had overbooked for Labor Day weekend, and if you weren't there thirty minutes before departure, your seat was awarded to the next traveler. There were no other flights to be had from San Francisco, and we needed to catch our return flight from Seattle to New York by noon the next day.

"I told you so," Elizabeth said smugly.

Lisette said, "I don't want to miss the first day of school."

I thought about the U.S. Open tickets we'd bought for Labor Day.

Gabriel took matters into his own hands. He booked the nearest available flight that would get us to Seattle on time. After staying on line at two rental car companies that were sold out, we finally found one remaining rental car. Gabriel drove through the night from San Francisco to Reno, Nevada. The girls slept in the back seat. Gabriel and I watched the shooting stars as we approached the bright lights of

Reno. We arrived at five a.m.—in time to make our morning flight to Seattle and then connect for the New York plane.

Gabriel and I did not develop a calm, uneventful life in the wake of IVF. I didn't board the cruise ship pregnant, as planned. But Gabriel and I did have each other. We would continue to face each situation together creatively. Gabriel was more accepting now that the girls could be difficult and still be part of his family. Elizabeth could not reconstruct the original family she had lost, but she was adjusting to this one and was a long way from her days of running off into the woods. Lisette was learning to balance time with her mother, stepfather, and family, and I in turn was less caught in the middle between Gabriel and the children. I now had faith in the longevity of our family. Over the past four years, without medical help, we had brought into existence a blended family that knew how to come together while each of us stayed true to our own nature.

Grade A Baby Eggs

Acknowledgments

I want to thank my family for their support and endurance of both my IVF trials and the writing of this memoir. Special thanks to Paul De Angelis for editing *Grade A Baby Eggs*, for helping me to make it shorter, and for his appreciation of my sense of humor. I want to express gratitude to Maura Shaw for her copyediting, her author support, and for providing positive feedback. The staff at Epigraph brought *Grade A Baby Eggs* into existence: Paul Cohen was enthusiastic from the beginning; Joe Tantillo used a creative and sensitive approach for the book design; and Tim Dillinger helped with the marketing. My memoir writing group, consisting of a greeting card illustrator, a psychologist, and a professor, gave me wonderful suggestions and fun times together. Thanks go to Lou Willett Stanek for her memoir-writing course at The New School and for listening to me read chapters from my book. Finally I also want to thank Philip Patrick and Penny Sansevieri for their insightful publishing courses at New York University.

Grade A Baby Eggs

Appendix

Cracking the Egg Donor Industry—Recommended Reforms

The world of egg donation is a Wild West free-for-all. There are no regulations and much exploitation. The seamier nature of my egg donor experience underlines the need for reform. Until ethical issues are addressed by either the industry or government regulation, egg donation is likely to remain an auction block for selling female flesh in the form of baby eggs, and donors will continue to be classified as Saks versus Wal-Mart and paid accordingly. The industry must provide safeguards for egg donors and treat them respectfully rather than as dispensable moneymakers. The popular donors become part of a "puppy mill" as they breed babies and risk death or their own subsequent infertility from multiple donations. One caring agency told me it would wait until after the donor's current donation to ask her if she wanted to donate again, let her process how she felt, and then honor her wishes. This attitude was in marked contrast to having donors cross state lines to allow for multiple donations and asking potential recipients to pay for a place on a huge waitlist. Early on, eBay took a stand by halting an online luxury auction of models' eggs and by outlawing all further egg sales.

When I was in the market for an egg, there was no real way of guaranteeing what egg I was getting. The facilities selling donor eggs need to obtain documentation from outside sources, such as diplomas and academic and job records, to verify the claims of the donor and/or agency promoting her.

Full disclosure of egg donation results by those marketing the donor, positive as well as negative, is imperative. Both the donor and the agency are motivated to report impregnations because "proven" donors charge higher prices. My second egg donor doctor informed me that some fertility operations retrieve unusable eggs anyway and add thousands more to the bill even when there is no chance of success. Fertility facilities need a protocol for when to discontinue doomed cycles.

It also is important to prevent price gouging. Prices vary greatly between hospitals, clinics, and agencies. On top of the price of the donor, some agencies charge a flat commission fee and others charge a percentage of the donor's rate. Charges must be made more uniform, and there should be monitoring to prevent exorbitant rates. A fertility legislative committee must consider ethical as well as financial factors when creating egg donor legislation.

Doctors working in this field should pay additional attention to the feelings of the fertility patient. It was shocking for me to be told at my first appointment to buy a donor egg. I did not consider my egg interchangeable with a donor's, and I had to embark on my own emotional journey before I could accept a donor egg; even then I was ambivalent about it. The factory-like atmosphere of the hospital should be addressed as well. Anxious potential mothers are not reassured when no one adequately explains procedures and when doctors rotate frequently and often remain nameless.

Infertile women wanting a baby are desperate. They will employ expensive methods with little hope of success and possible threats to their safety and that of their hoped-for baby. I myself tried IVF five times with a single-digit chance of its working. I also hoped to attempt the risky, outlawed splicing of my egg with a younger egg that could have resulted in a Frankenstein baby with too many genes. Women need to be made aware of the odds that they are facing and the benefits and risks of each procedure. The vignette of the doctor who wears a top hat and waves a magic wand over the abdomen of his fertility patient provides an apt metaphor for the hocus pocus that is involved in much of the fertility process.

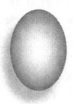

Readers' Discussion Guide

1. Victoria already had two children and Gabriel had none. Do you think they shared the same goals for having a baby? How did their priorities overlap? How did they differ?

2. From the beginning Elizabeth and Lisette did not want a new sibling—only a puppy. How did the years of medical baby making affect them? Do you think that their attitude toward having an infant in the family changed over time?

3. The practice of IVF has enormous emotional and financial costs and calls for a significant time commitment. Were you surprised by what the process of IVF entails and how it becomes so consuming for its participants?

4. Victoria often felt isolated during the IVF process. Do you think that there should be more opportunities for support among the women undergoing fertility treatments?

5. Infertility is a hot topic in the media. Movies such as *Baby Mama*, *The Switch*, *The Back-up Plan* and *The Kids Are All Right* tackle topics such as surrogacy and sperm donation. How do the concerns of the characters in these films overlap with and differ from those confronted by Gabriel and Victoria?

6. Women's eggs are bought and sold over the internet. Some women's eggs are worth more than others. Women with high SAT scores who look like models and had a successful prior donation command the highest prices. What do you think about the donor

egg market? If you were purchasing eggs, would you shop for certain characteristics?

7. What are the ethical issues raised by egg donation? In some countries, such as Australia, it is illegal to pay the egg donor. Do you think that women should be reimbursed for donating their eggs in the United States? If so, should there be laws to limit the amount of payment?

8. Gabriel was ready to use donor eggs from the start, and Victoria was adamantly opposed. How did she journey toward acceptance of utilizing an egg donor, and why was she still ambivalent? What are the similarities and differences between using donor eggs and adopting?

9. There is a stigma attached to egg donation. Victoria found that one of the hospitals did not run any egg donor recipient support groups so that women could keep the origin of their babies a secret. She also was informed that women want to match their blood type to their egg donor so that they never have to reveal to their children that they are not the biological mothers. Do you think that women should be more open about egg donation? Would you tell your own child if you used a donor egg?

10. Gabriel and Victoria tried IVF five times with Victoria's eggs, and they attempted egg donation twice. Will Victoria keep looking for new advances and try again? In the meantime what sort of resolution have they achieved with their inability to conceive?